The PCOS Kitchen Makeover: *Mediterranean Healing Recipes*

Dominic Marsh

Table of Contents

Chapter 1: Introduction To PCOS And The Mediterranean Diet:

Polycystic Ovary Syndrome (PCOS) is a common hormonal disorder that affects individuals with reproductive systems. It's characterized by irregular periods, elevated levels of androgens (male hormones), and the development of small cysts on the ovaries. PCOS can lead to a range of symptoms, including weight gain, insulin resistance, acne, and fertility issues.

The Mediterranean Diet, on the other hand, is a dietary pattern inspired by the traditional eating habits of countries bordering the Mediterranean Sea. It's renowned for its health benefits and has been linked to a reduced risk of heart disease, diabetes, and even certain cancers. The diet is centered around whole, minimally processed foods that are rich in nutrients and antioxidants.

The synergy between PCOS management and the Mediterranean Diet lies in its emphasis on whole foods, healthy fats, lean proteins, and complex carbohydrates. This approach can help address some of the underlying issues associated with PCOS, such as insulin resistance and inflammation.

By adopting the Mediterranean Diet, individuals with PCOS can potentially experience improved insulin sensitivity, better weight management, and reduced inflammation. The diet's incorporation of nutrient-dense foods can also support hormone balance and overall well-being.

In this cookbook, we explore the intersection of PCOS and the Mediterranean Diet, providing you with a collection of delicious and nourishing recipes. From breakfast to dinner, and even delectable desserts, you'll discover flavorful ways to support your PCOS journey while enjoying the culinary delights of the Mediterranean region.

Understanding PCOS and Its Impact on Health:

Polycystic Ovary Syndrome (PCOS) is a complex hormonal disorder that affects individuals with ovaries, often during their reproductive years. It's a condition characterized by various hormonal imbalances and physical symptoms that can impact overall health and well-being. Let's delve into some key aspects of PCOS and its effects on health:

i. **Hormonal Imbalance**: One of the hallmarks of PCOS is an elevated level of androgens, commonly referred to as "male hormones." This imbalance can lead to a range of symptoms, including irregular or absent menstrual cycles, excess hair growth (hirsutism), and acne.

ii. **Insulin Resistance**: Many individuals with PCOS experience insulin resistance, a condition in which the body's cells do not respond effectively to insulin. This can lead to elevated blood sugar levels and an increased risk of type 2 diabetes.

iii. **Weight Gain**: Insulin resistance can contribute to weight gain, and excess weight can further exacerbate insulin resistance. This creates a cycle that can be challenging to break and may impact overall metabolic health.

iv. **Fertility Challenges**: PCOS is a leading cause of infertility due to irregular ovulation or lack of ovulation. Hormonal imbalances can disrupt the normal menstrual cycle and hinder the release of mature eggs.

v. **Cardiovascular Health**: Women with PCOS may have an increased risk of cardiovascular issues, including high blood pressure, high cholesterol levels, and an increased likelihood of developing heart disease.

vi.   **Mental Health**: PCOS is also linked to mental health concerns. The hormonal fluctuations, physical symptoms, and challenges related to fertility can contribute to anxiety, depression, and a reduced quality of life.

vii.   **Inflammation**: Chronic low-grade inflammation is often observed in individuals with PCOS. This inflammation can contribute to various health problems, including insulin resistance and cardiovascular issues.

Managing PCOS involves a holistic approach that addresses the underlying hormonal imbalances, insulin resistance, and other associated health concerns. Lifestyle modifications, including a balanced diet, regular exercise, stress management, and potentially medication, can play a crucial role in improving symptoms and overall well-being.

The Mediterranean Diet, with its focus on whole, nutrient-rich foods, can be particularly beneficial for individuals with PCOS. Its emphasis on anti-inflammatory foods, healthy fats, and complex carbohydrates aligns well with the goals of managing PCOS symptoms and promoting better health outcomes. This cookbook aims to guide you through the journey of combining the benefits of the Mediterranean Diet with PCOS management for a more vibrant and balanced life.

1.2 The principles and benefits of the Mediterranean diet

The Mediterranean Diet is a dietary pattern inspired by the traditional eating habits of countries bordering the Mediterranean Sea, such as Greece, Italy, and Spain. It's renowned for its health benefits and has gained popularity worldwide. Here are the key principles and benefits of the Mediterranean Diet:

i. Principles of the Mediterranean Diet:

- **Plant-Centric**: The diet is centered around plant-based foods such as fruits, vegetables, whole grains, legumes, nuts, and seeds. These foods are rich in vitamins, minerals, fiber, and antioxidants.

- **Healthy Fats**: The diet emphasizes healthy fats, particularly monounsaturated fats found in olive oil. These fats are associated with heart health and can help reduce the risk of chronic diseases.

- **Lean Proteins**: Fish and poultry are preferred over red meat. Fish, especially fatty fish like salmon and sardines, are rich in omega-3 fatty acids that support heart and brain health.

- **Moderate Dairy**: Moderate consumption of dairy products, such as yogurt and cheese, is part of the diet. These provide calcium and probiotics for gut health.

- **Red Wine in Moderation**: Some versions of the diet include moderate consumption of red wine, which is thought to have heart-protective effects due to its antioxidant content.

- **Whole Grains**: Whole grains like whole wheat, brown rice, and quinoa provide sustained energy and are rich in fiber, which supports digestive health.

- **Fresh Herbs and Spices**: Flavor is derived from herbs and spices rather than excessive salt. This adds variety and provides potential health benefits.

- **Social and Active Lifestyle**: The Mediterranean
  Diet is often enjoyed in the company of others
  and encourages regular physical activity.

- **Heart Health**: The diet's emphasis on healthy
  fats, such as olive oil and nuts, can improve
  cholesterol levels and reduce the risk of heart
  disease.

- **Weight Management**: The diet's focus on whole
  foods and portion control can contribute to
  weight loss and maintenance.

- **Reduced Risk of Chronic Diseases**: The
  Mediterranean Diet has been linked to a lower
  risk of type 2 diabetes, certain cancers, and
  neurodegenerative diseases like Alzheimer's.

- **Improved Brain Health**: The consumption of
  omega-3 fatty acids from fish and antioxidants
  from fruits and vegetables supports cognitive
  function and may reduce the risk of cognitive
  decline.

- **Better Blood Sugar Control**: The diet's emphasis on whole grains and fiber-rich foods can help regulate blood sugar levels.

- **Anti-Inflammatory Effects**: The diet's abundant plant-based foods and healthy fats have anti-inflammatory properties that can help reduce inflammation in the body.

- **Longevity**: Studies suggest that adherence to the Mediterranean Diet is associated with a longer life and a lower risk of premature death.

- **Digestive Health**: The fiber from fruits, vegetables, and whole grains supports a healthy gut and can aid digestion.

By incorporating the principles of the Mediterranean Diet into your eating habits, you can enjoy a balanced and flavorful way of eating that offers a wide range of health benefits, from cardiovascular well-being to improved overall longevity.

1.3 How this cookbook can help manage PCOS symptoms

This cookbook is designed to be a valuable resource for individuals managing PCOS by combining the principles of the Mediterranean Diet with specific strategies to address PCOS symptoms. Here's how this cookbook can aid in managing PCOS symptoms:

- **Balanced Nutrition**: The Mediterranean Diet's emphasis on whole foods, lean proteins, healthy fats, and complex carbohydrates aligns well with the nutritional needs of individuals with PCOS. By following the recipes in this cookbook, you'll be consuming nutrient-dense meals that can help regulate blood sugar levels and support hormone balance.

- **Controlled Insulin Levels**: Many recipes in the cookbook focus on foods with a low glycemic index, which helps prevent rapid spikes in blood sugar. This is particularly important for individuals with PCOS and insulin resistance.

- **Anti-Inflammatory Foods**: The Mediterranean Diet is rich in anti-inflammatory foods, such as fruits, vegetables, and fatty fish. Inflammation is often a factor in PCOS, and consuming these foods can help reduce overall inflammation in the body.

- **Heart Health**: PCOS is associated with an increased risk of cardiovascular issues. The

Mediterranean Diet's inclusion of heart-healthy fats like olive oil, along with omega-3 fatty acids from fish, can support cardiovascular well-being.

- **Weight Management**: Many individuals with PCOS struggle with weight management. The balanced approach of the Mediterranean Diet, along with portion control and whole foods, can contribute to healthy weight loss and maintenance.

- **Fertility Support**: By providing essential nutrients and supporting hormone balance, the recipes in this cookbook can aid in regulating menstrual cycles and improving fertility for those trying to conceive.

- **Stress Reduction**: Stress can exacerbate PCOS symptoms. The Mediterranean Diet's focus on social connections and stress-reducing activities aligns with the holistic approach to PCOS management.

- **Digestive Health**: The fiber-rich foods in the diet can support gut health and digestion, which are crucial for overall well-being.

- **Improved Mental Health**: The incorporation of nutrient-rich foods and healthy fats can positively impact mood and mental well-being, which can be particularly important for individuals dealing with PCOS-related emotional challenges.

- **Long-Term Lifestyle**: The Mediterranean Diet isn't a quick-fix solution; it's a sustainable lifestyle. By adopting these eating habits, you're creating a foundation for long-term health and symptom management.

Ultimately, this cookbook offers a comprehensive approach to PCOS management by combining the principles of the Mediterranean Diet with considerations specific to PCOS symptoms. The flavorful and diverse recipes make it easier and more enjoyable to adhere to a dietary plan that supports your well-being and helps you thrive while managing PCOS.

Chapter 2: Mediterranean Pantry Staples

Creating a Mediterranean-inspired pantry is key to successfully following the diet. Here's a list of essential Mediterranean pantry staples that can serve as the foundation for your PCOS-friendly meals:

- **Extra Virgin Olive Oil**: A cornerstone of the Mediterranean Diet, rich in healthy monounsaturated fats and antioxidants.

- **Whole Grains**: Stock up on quinoa, brown rice, whole wheat pasta, bulgur, and farro for wholesome carbohydrate options.

- **Legumes**: Include lentils, chickpeas, black beans, and cannellini beans as excellent sources of plant-based protein and fiber.

- **Nuts and Seeds**: Almonds, walnuts, flaxseeds, and chia seeds provide healthy fats, protein, and nutrients for your meals.

- **Herbs and Spices**: Herbs like basil, oregano, rosemary, and thyme, along with spices like cumin, paprika, and turmeric, add depth and flavor to dishes.

- **Canned Tomatoes**: Tomatoes and tomato products like diced tomatoes, tomato paste, and tomato sauce are essential for Mediterranean cooking.

- **Fish and Seafood**: Opt for canned tuna, salmon, and sardines packed in olive oil or water, as well as frozen fish fillets.

- **Poultry and Lean Meats**: While not as prominent as other sources of protein, having lean cuts of chicken and turkey can be useful.

- **Dairy and Dairy Alternatives**: Greek yogurt, feta cheese, and unsweetened almond or coconut milk are common choices.

- **Fresh Produce**: Load up on a variety of fresh vegetables like tomatoes, cucumbers, bell peppers, leafy greens, and zucchini.

- **Fruits**: Keep fruits like berries, citrus fruits, apples, and pears on hand for snacking and meal accompaniments.

- **Whole Wheat Flour**: If you enjoy baking, opt for whole wheat flour for a healthier twist on baked goods.

- **Whole Wheat Bread**: Choose whole grain bread for sandwiches and toast.

- **Eggs**: A versatile source of protein that can be used in various Mediterranean-inspired dishes.

- **Olives**: A staple in Mediterranean cuisine, olives provide flavor and healthy fats.

- **Onions and Garlic**: These aromatic vegetables are used as a base for many Mediterranean dishes.

- **Vinegars**: Balsamic vinegar, red wine vinegar, and apple cider vinegar are great for dressings and marinades.

- **Dark Chocolate**: For an occasional treat, opt for dark chocolate with a high cocoa content.

- **Herbal Teas**: Herbal teas like chamomile and mint are soothing and align with the Mediterranean's emphasis on natural ingredients.

- **Dried Fruits**: In moderation, dried fruits like raisins, apricots, and dates can be used to add natural sweetness to recipes.

By keeping these Mediterranean pantry staples on hand, you'll be well-equipped to create a variety of PCOS-friendly meals that are not only delicious but also supportive of your health and well-being.

2.1 Essential ingredients for a PCOS-friendly Mediterranean kitchen

Creating a PCOS-friendly Mediterranean kitchen involves incorporating foods that align with both the Mediterranean Diet and the specific needs of individuals managing PCOS. Here are essential ingredients to have in your PCOS-friendly Mediterranean kitchen:

a) Extra Virgin Olive Oil: A cornerstone of the Mediterranean Diet, it is rich in monounsaturated fats and antioxidants that support heart health and hormone balance.

b) Whole Grains: Opt for whole grains like quinoa, brown rice, whole wheat pasta, and oats. These provide complex carbohydrates and fiber that regulate blood sugar levels.

c) Legumes: Lentils, chickpeas, black beans, and other legumes are excellent sources of plant-based protein, fiber, and essential nutrients.

d) Fatty Fish: Incorporate fatty fish like salmon, mackerel, and sardines for their omega-3 fatty acids, which have anti-inflammatory effects and support hormone regulation.

e) Lean Proteins: Include lean poultry (chicken, turkey) and lean cuts of meat in moderation for a balanced protein intake.

f) Nuts and Seeds: Almonds, walnuts, flaxseeds, chia seeds, and pumpkin seeds provide healthy fats, fiber, and essential nutrients.

g) Fresh Produce: Stock up on a variety of colorful vegetables (leafy greens, bell peppers, tomatoes and zucchini) and fruits (berries, citrus, apples and pears) for vitamins, minerals, and antioxidants.

h) Herbs and Spices: Utilize herbs like basil, oregano, rosemary, and spices such as cumin and turmeric to enhance flavors without excessive salt.

i) Greek Yogurt: A protein-rich dairy option that can be used as a base for creamy dressings, dips, and smoothies.

j) Feta Cheese: In moderation, feta cheese adds a burst of flavor to salads, omelets, and various Mediterranean dishes.

k) Tomato Products: Canned tomatoes, tomato paste, and tomato sauce are versatile ingredients for sauces and stews.

l) Onions and Garlic: These aromatic vegetables add depth and flavor to your dishes and have potential health benefits.

m) Vinegars: Balsamic vinegar, red wine vinegar, and apple cider vinegar are essential for creating flavorful dressings and marinades.

n) Whole Wheat Flour: If you enjoy baking, opt for whole wheat flour to make PCOS-friendly baked goods.

o) Herbal Teas: Chamomile, mint, and other herbal teas can provide soothing and calming effects.

p) Dark Chocolate: In moderation, dark chocolate with a high cocoa content can satisfy sweet cravings without excessive sugar.

q) Herbal Supplements: Consult your healthcare provider about incorporating supplements like inositol, which has shown potential benefits for PCOS management.

By combining these PCOS-friendly ingredients with the principles of the Mediterranean Diet, you can create nourishing and flavorful meals that support your health and well-being while managing PCOS symptoms.

2.2 Tips for sourcing and storing ingredients:

Sourcing and storing ingredients effectively is crucial for maintaining a PCOS-friendly Mediterranean kitchen. Here are some tips to help you with these tasks:

1. Sourcing Ingredients:

i) Local Markets: Explore local farmers' markets for fresh, seasonal produce. Locally sourced items often have better flavor and nutritional value.

ii) Grocery Stores: Choose stores with a wide selection of whole foods, organic options, and lean proteins. Read labels to ensure you're selecting minimally processed options.

iii) Online Shopping: Consider online grocery delivery services, which can be convenient for busy schedules. Look for websites that specialize in organic or health-focused products.

iv) Bulk Buying: Purchase staple items like whole grains, legumes, and nuts in bulk. This can save money and reduce packaging waste.

v) Fish Markets: For fresh seafood, visit local fish markets to find high-quality, sustainable options.

vi) Specialty Stores: Explore specialty stores that offer Mediterranean ingredients like olive oil, spices, and cheeses.

2. Storing Ingredients:

i) Refrigeration: Keep perishable items like fresh produce, dairy, and lean proteins in the refrigerator at the appropriate temperatures.

ii) Freezing: If you buy in bulk or want to extend the shelf life of certain items, freezing is a great option. Portion items like berries or fish fillets before freezing for easier use.

iii) Airtight Containers: Store dry goods like whole grains, nuts, and seeds in airtight containers to maintain freshness and prevent moisture.

iv) Labeling: Label containers with the purchase or expiration date to ensure you use items before they spoil.

v) First In, First Out (FIFO): When storing items, place newer purchases behind older ones to use up older ingredients first.

vi) Herbs and Greens: Store fresh herbs in a glass of water or wrapped in a damp paper towel inside a plastic bag in the refrigerator. Use airtight containers or produce storage bags for leafy greens to prevent wilting.

vii) Spices: Store spices in a cool, dark place away from direct sunlight to preserve their flavors.

viii) Olive Oil: Store olive oil in a cool, dark place and tightly seal the bottle to prevent exposure to air and light, which can cause it to go rancid.

ix) Tomato Products: Once opened, transfer canned tomato products to a glass or plastic container with a tight-fitting lid and store in the refrigerator.

x) Clear Visibility: Organize your pantry and refrigerator to allow for clear visibility of ingredients. This makes it easier to find what you need and prevents items from getting forgotten.

By sourcing fresh and quality ingredients and practicing proper storage techniques, you'll ensure that your PCOS-friendly Mediterranean kitchen is well-stocked with items that promote your health and well-being.

Chapter 3: Breakfast Delights

Certainly! Here are some Mediterranean-inspired breakfast ideas that are not only delicious but also PCOS-friendly:

- **Mediterranean Veggie Omelet**: Whisk together eggs or egg whites with chopped bell peppers, tomatoes, spinach, and a sprinkle of feta cheese. Cook in olive oil for a flavorful and nutrient-packed omelet.

- **Greek Yogurt Parfait**: Layer Greek yogurt with fresh berries, chopped nuts, and a drizzle of honey for a protein-rich and satisfying breakfast.

- **Mediterranean Avocado Toast**: Top whole grain toast with smashed avocado, sliced tomatoes, a sprinkle of feta cheese, and a drizzle of olive oil. Add a poached egg for extra protein.

- **Mediterranean Smoothie**: Blend together frozen berries, a handful of spinach, Greek yogurt, a splash of almond milk, and a tablespoon of chia seeds for a nutrient-dense smoothie.

- **Smoked Salmon Breakfast Wrap**: Fill a whole wheat tortilla with smoked salmon, cucumber slices, red onion, and a dollop of Greek yogurt mixed with dill.

- o **Homemade Granola Bowl**: Create a bowl with your homemade granola (oats, nuts, seeds, and a touch of honey), topped with Greek yogurt and fresh fruit.

- o **Mediterranean Quinoa Bowl**: Cook quinoa and top it with sautéed spinach, roasted cherry tomatoes, olives, and a sprinkle of feta cheese.

- o **Egg and Veggie Breakfast Burrito**: Scramble eggs with sautéed bell peppers, onions, and a handful of spinach. Wrap the mixture in a whole wheat tortilla.

- o **Mediterranean Frittata**: Mix eggs with diced tomatoes, bell peppers, red onion, and chopped olives. Bake until set, and enjoy slices of this hearty frittata.

- o **Chia Seed Pudding**: Make a chia seed pudding using almond milk, chia seeds, and a touch of honey. Top with fresh berries and chopped nuts.

Remember, the key to a PCOS-friendly breakfast is to focus on whole foods, lean proteins, and healthy fats to support blood sugar regulation and hormone balance.

These breakfast ideas provide a great starting point for a delicious and nutritious morning meal.

3.1 Nutrient-packed breakfast recipes to kickstart your day

Absolutely! Here are some nutrient-packed breakfast recipes that can help you kickstart your day on a healthy note:

1. Berry Nut Smoothie Bowl:

- Blend frozen mixed berries, a banana, Greek yogurt, and a splash of almond milk until smooth.
- Pour into a bowl and top with sliced almonds, chia seeds, and fresh berries.

2. Spinach and Feta Breakfast Wrap:

- Sauté spinach and cherry tomatoes in olive oil until wilted.
- Beat eggs, pour into the pan, and scramble with the vegetables.
- Fill a whole wheat tortilla with the scrambled mixture, crumbled feta cheese, and a sprinkle of chopped fresh herbs.

3. Mediterranean Breakfast Salad:

- o Combine chopped cucumbers, tomatoes, red onion, bell peppers, and olives.
- o Toss with extra virgin olive oil, lemon juice, and chopped fresh parsley.
- o Top with crumbled feta cheese and a poached egg.

4. Quinoa and Fruit Breakfast Bowl:

- o Cook quinoa and let it cool. Mix with diced mango, kiwi, and pomegranate seeds.
- o Drizzle with a touch of honey and sprinkle with chopped nuts and seeds.

5. Sweet Potato and Black Bean Hash:

- o Sauté diced sweet potatoes, black beans, and bell peppers in olive oil.
- o Season with cumin, paprika, and a pinch of red pepper flakes.
- o Top with a fried egg and a dollop of Greek yogurt.

6. Avocado and Egg Breakfast Toast:

- o Mash avocado onto whole-grain toast.
- o Top with a poached or fried egg, a sprinkle of chili flakes, and a drizzle of olive oil.

7. Mediterranean Yogurt Parfait:

o   Layer Greek yogurt with diced cucumbers, tomatoes, and red onion.
o   Top with Kalamata olives, a sprinkle of za'atar spice, and a drizzle of olive oil.

8. Oatmeal with Nuts and Seeds:

o   Cook oats with almond milk and a touch of cinnamon.
o   Top with chopped nuts, chia seeds, and a handful of mixed berries.

9. Veggie and Hummus Breakfast Wrap:

o   Spread hummus on a whole- wheat tortilla.
o   Fill with sautéed spinach, roasted red peppers, and scrambled eggs.

10. Salmon and Asparagus Breakfast Plate:

o   Grill or bake salmon fillets and asparagus spears.
o   Serve with whole- grain toast, a side of Greek yogurt, and lemon wedges.

These recipes are loaded with nutrients, including fiber, protein, healthy fats, vitamins, and minerals, which are perfect for starting your day with energy and nourishment while managing PCOS.

3.2 Mediterranean-inspired smoothies, omelets, and grain bowls

Here are some Mediterranean-inspired recipes for smoothies, omelets, and grain bowls:

i. Mediterranean-Inspired Smoothie:

- o Blend together 1 cup of spinach, 1/2 cup of frozen mixed berries, 1/4 cup of Greek yogurt, 1 tablespoon of chia seeds, 1 teaspoon of honey, and a splash of almond milk.
- o Add a sprinkle of ground flaxseeds and a few chopped walnuts on top.

ii. Mediterranean Vegetable Omelet:

- o Whisk together 2-3 eggs with a splash of almond milk, salt, and pepper.
- o In a skillet, sauté diced bell peppers, red onion, and cherry tomatoes in olive oil until softened.
- o Pour the egg mixture over the vegetables and cook until set. Sprinkle with crumbled feta cheese and chopped fresh herbs before folding the omelet in half.

iii. Mediterranean Quinoa Grain Bowl:

- o Cook the quinoa according to the package instructions and let it cool slightly.

- o Arrange the quinoa in a bowl and top with cooked and cooled chickpeas, sliced cucumber, chopped Kalamata olives, diced red onion, and crumbled feta cheese.
- o Drizzle with a dressing made from extra virgin olive oil, lemon juice, minced garlic, and dried oregano.

iv. Mediterranean Breakfast Smoothie Bowl:

- o Blend together 1 frozen banana, 1/2 cup of Greek yogurt, a handful of spinach, 1 tablespoon of almond butter, and a splash of almond milk until creamy.
- o Pour the smoothie into a bowl and top with sliced strawberries, crushed pistachios, and a sprinkle of shredded coconut.

v. Greek-Inspired Omelet Wrap:

- o In a bowl, beat two eggs with a pinch of dried oregano and a dash of black pepper.
- o Pour the mixture into a heated non-stick skillet and cook until almost set.
- o Add diced tomatoes, crumbled feta cheese, and chopped fresh parsley to one side of the omelet.
- o Fold the other side over the filling and cook for another minute until the cheese melts.

vi. Mediterranean Farro Bowl:

- o   Cook farro according to package instructions.
- o   Toss cooked farro with roasted red peppers, artichoke hearts, cooked and cooled shrimp, and diced cucumber.
- o   Drizzle with a lemon and olive oil vinaigrette, and top with chopped fresh dill.

These Mediterranean-inspired recipes for smoothies, omelets, and grain bowls combine the flavors and ingredients of the Mediterranean Diet with creative twists for a satisfying and nourishing breakfast experience.

Chapter 4: Wholesome Appetizers And Snacks

Here are some wholesome Mediterranean-inspired appetizers and snacks that are not only delicious but also suitable for managing PCOS:

1. Wholesome Appetizers:

- o **Hummus and Veggie Platter**: Serve homemade hummus with an array of colorful vegetable sticks such as carrots, cucumbers, bell peppers, and cherry tomatoes.

- o **Stuffed Grape Leaves**: Fill grape leaves with a mixture of cooked quinoa, chopped fresh herbs, diced tomatoes, and a drizzle of olive oil.

- o **Greek Salad Skewers**: Thread cherry tomatoes, cucumber cubes, olives, and feta cheese onto small skewers. Drizzle with olive oil and sprinkle with oregano.

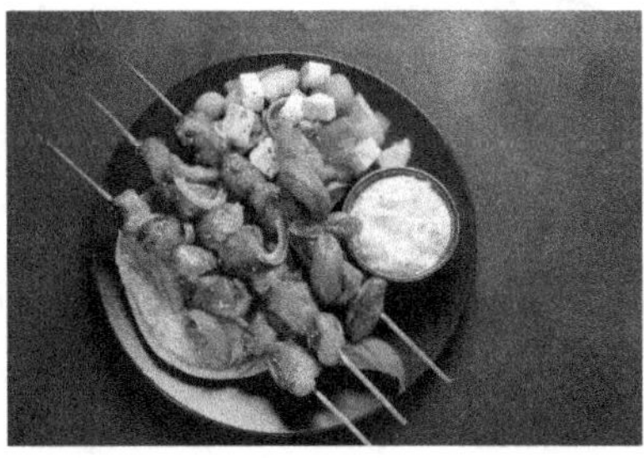

Fried Souvlaki, Greek Salad and tzatziki

o **Spinach and Feta Stuffed Mushrooms**: Fill
button mushroom caps with a mixture of sautéed
spinach, crumbled feta, and garlic. Bake until the
mushrooms are tender.

o **Zucchini Fritters**: Grate zucchini and mix it
with chopped fresh mint, crumbled feta, and an
egg. Shape into small patties and cook until
golden.

2. Wholesome Snacks:

o **Greek Yogurt with Berries**: Enjoy a serving of
Greek yogurt topped with a mix of fresh berries
and a sprinkle of chopped nuts.

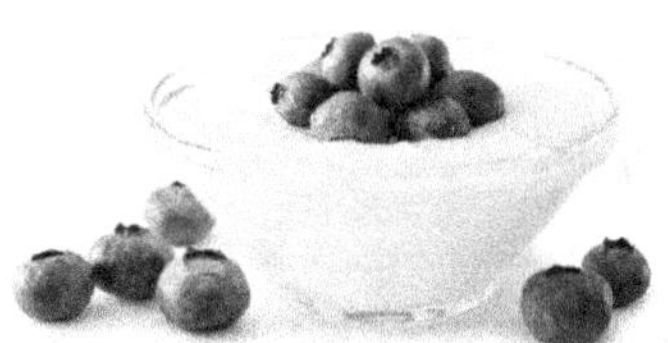

Bowl of Greek Yoghurt with blue berries

o **Mixed Nuts and Seeds**: Create your own trail mix with a variety of nuts like almonds, walnuts, and pistachios, along with seeds like pumpkin and sunflower.

o **Roasted Chickpeas**: Toss cooked chickpeas with olive oil and your favorite spices. Roast until crispy for a satisfying, crunchy snack.

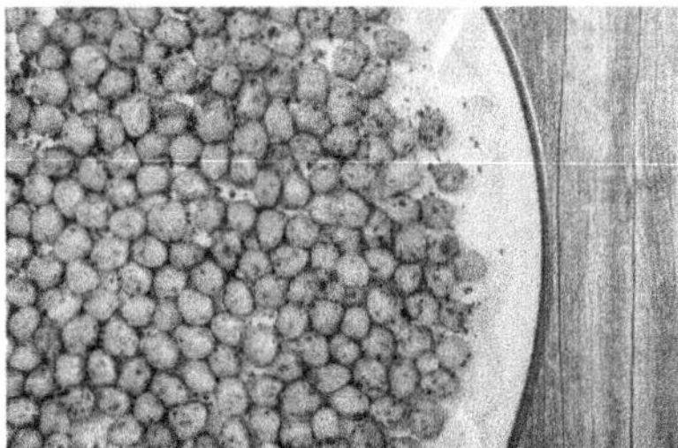

Roasted Spicy Snack Chickpeas

o **Olive Tapenade on Whole Wheat Crackers**: Spread olive tapenade on whole wheat crackers or slices of cucumber for a flavorful snack.

o **Fruit and Cheese**: Pair slices of apple or pear with slices of cheese, such as feta or goat cheese, for a balanced sweet and savory snack.

o   **Crispy Kale Chips**: Coat kale leaves with a touch of olive oil and bake until crispy for a nutrient-rich snack.

Remember to focus on portion control while enjoying these appetizers and snacks, as moderation is key to maintaining a balanced diet while managing PCOS. These options provide a mix of fiber, protein, and healthy fats to keep you satisfied and energized throughout the day.

4.1 Tasty and healthy bites perfect for any occasion

Here are some tasty and healthy Mediterranean-inspired bites that are perfect for any occasion:

i. Mediterranean Bruschetta:

Top whole-grain baguette slices with diced tomatoes, minced garlic, chopped fresh basil, and a drizzle of balsamic vinegar.

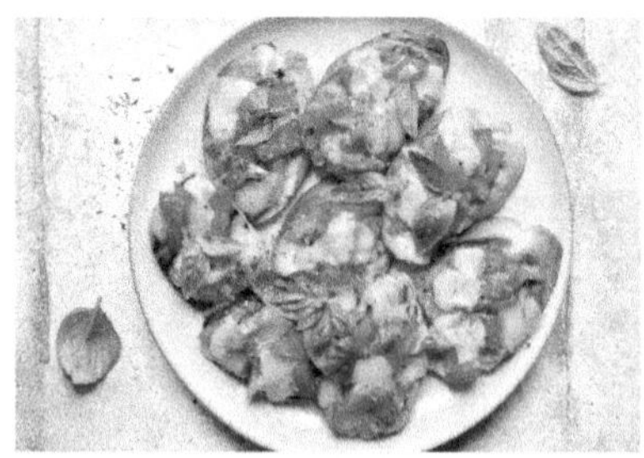

Grilled Bruschetta with tomato and mozzarela

ii. Cucumber and Greek Yogurt Dip:

Mix Greek yogurt with finely chopped cucumber, minced garlic, dill, lemon juice, and a pinch of salt. Serve with whole wheat pita chips or vegetable sticks.

iii. Mediterranean Deviled Eggs:

Make deviled eggs with mashed avocado, a dash of lemon juice, chopped Kalamata olives, and a sprinkle of paprika.

iv. Mediterranean Stuffed Mini Peppers:

Fill mini bell peppers with a mixture of cooked quinoa, black beans, corn, diced tomatoes, and feta cheese. Bake until the peppers are tender.

v. Olive and Cheese Skewers:

Thread Kalamata olives, cubes of feta cheese, and cherry tomatoes onto small skewers. Drizzle with olive oil and sprinkle with oregano.

vi. Spinach and Feta Phyllo Cups:

Fill mini phyllo cups with a mixture of sautéed spinach, crumbled feta, and a touch of nutmeg. Bake until golden.

vii. Mediterranean Cucumber Cups:

Scoop out the cucumber halves to create cups. Fill with a mixture of diced tomatoes, red onion, chopped mint, and crumbled goat cheese.

viii. Herbed Chickpea Salad in Endive Leaves:

Mix chickpeas with chopped fresh herbs, diced cucumber, lemon juice, and olive oil. Spoon the mixture into the endive leaves.

ix. Zucchini Roll-Ups:

Use thinly sliced zucchini as wraps. Fill with hummus, roasted red peppers, and a sprinkle of pine nuts. Roll up and secure with toothpicks.

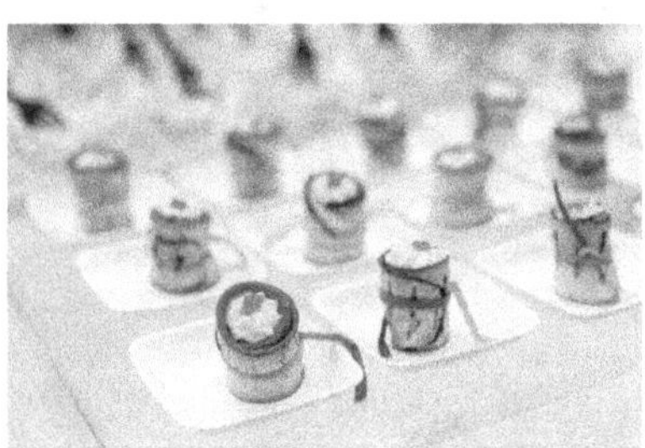

Bite-sized Grilled Zucchini Roll-ups for appetizer

x. Mediterranean Quinoa Bites:

Combine cooked quinoa with chopped spinach, diced tomatoes, chopped olives, and crumbled feta. Shape into bite-sized patties and bake until golden.

These bite-sized appetizers are not only visually appealing but also packed with Mediterranean flavors and nutrients. They're perfect for parties, gatherings, or simply enjoying healthy snacks.

4.2 Hummus variations, stuffed veggies, and more

Absolutely, let's explore some creative hummus variations, stuffed vegetable ideas, and a few additional Mediterranean-inspired bites:

1. Hummus Variations:

- **Roasted Red Pepper Hummus:**Blend roasted red bell peppers with chickpeas, tahini, garlic, lemon juice, and olive oil for a smoky and slightly sweet hummus.

- **Sun-Dried Tomato Hummus**: Add sun-dried tomatoes, basil leaves, pine nuts, and a dash of

balsamic vinegar to your hummus for a rich and
tangy flavor.

o   **Spinach and Artichoke Hummus**: Mix chopped
spinach, artichoke hearts, and a touch of
Parmesan cheese into hummus for a creamy and
savory twist.

o   **Beet Hummus**: Blend cooked beets with
chickpeas, tahini, lemon juice, and a pinch of
cumin for a vibrant and earthy hummus.

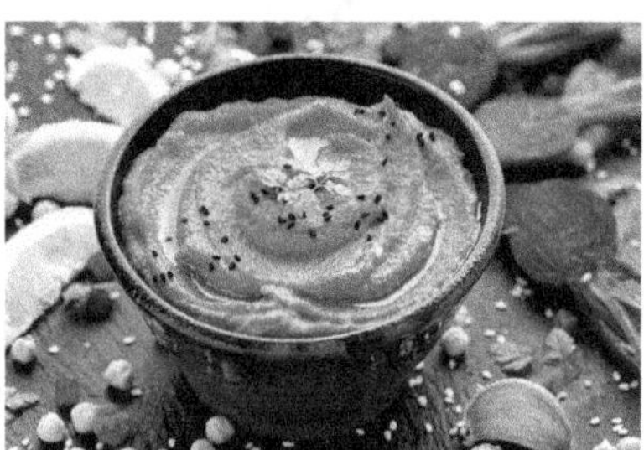

Roasted Beet Hummus

o   **Olive Tapenade Hummus**: Incorporate
Kalamata olives, capers, and a drizzle of olive oil
into hummus for a briny and intense flavor
profile.

2. Stuffed Vegetable Ideas:

o **Stuffed Bell Peppers**: Fill halved bell peppers with a mixture of cooked quinoa, lean ground turkey, diced tomatoes, chopped herbs, and feta cheese. Bake until the peppers are tender.

o **Stuffed Portobello Mushrooms**: Stuff Portobello mushroom caps with a mixture of sautéed spinach, cooked brown rice, diced tomatoes, and grated Parmesan cheese. Bake until mushrooms are cooked through.

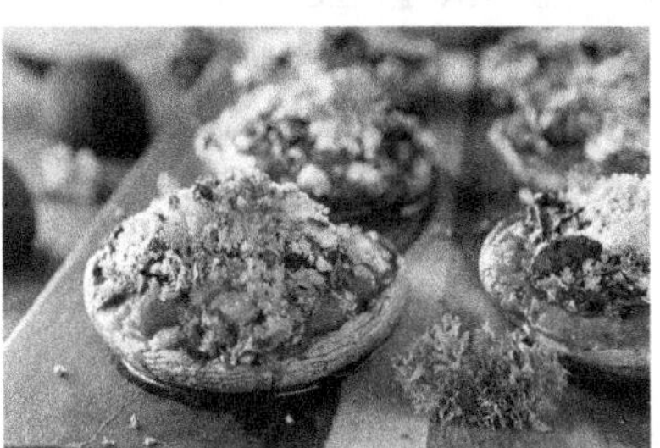

Homemade Stuffed Portobello Mushrooms

o **Stuffed Zucchini Boats**: Hollow out zucchini halves and fill with a mixture of cooked lentils, diced bell peppers, red onion, and crumbled goat cheese. Bake until the zucchini is tender.

4.3 Additional Mediterranean-Inspired Bites:

- o **Mediterranean Sushi Rolls**: Fill nori sheets with hummus, sliced cucumber, roasted red peppers, and avocado. Roll tightly and slice into bite-sized pieces.

- o **Caprese Skewers**: Thread cherry tomatoes, fresh mozzarella balls, and basil leaves onto skewers. Drizzle with balsamic glaze.

- o **Crispy Eggplant Rounds**: Coat thin eggplant slices with whole wheat breadcrumbs and bake until crispy. Top with tomato slices, mozzarella, and fresh basil.

- o **Za'atar Pita Chips**: Cut whole wheat pita bread into triangles, brush with olive oil, and sprinkle with za'atar spice. Bake until crispy.

- o **Mediterranean Stuffed Dates**: Fill pitted dates with a mixture of goat cheese and chopped nuts, then drizzle with honey.

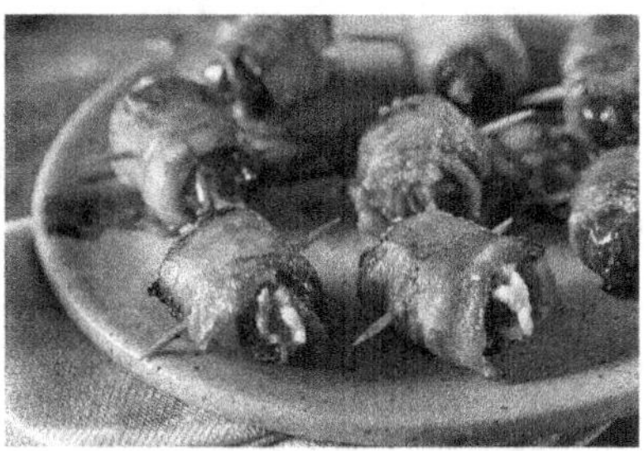

Homemade Stuffed Dates

These variations and ideas offer a wide range of flavors and textures, making them perfect for entertaining, snacking, or even light meals. They embrace the rich and diverse flavors of the Mediterranean while providing nutritious options for a balanced diet.

Chapter 5: Fresh Salads and Dressings

Here are some fresh Mediterranean-inspired salad ideas, along with homemade dressing recipes to complement them:

- **Greek Salad**: Toss together chopped cucumbers, tomatoes, red onion, Kalamata olives, and crumbled feta cheese. Sprinkle with dried oregano and drizzle with extra virgin olive oil and lemon juice.

- **Mediterranean Chickpea Salad**: Combine cooked chickpeas with diced cucumber, red bell pepper, red onion, cherry tomatoes, chopped parsley, and crumbled feta. Toss with a lemon-oregano vinaigrette.

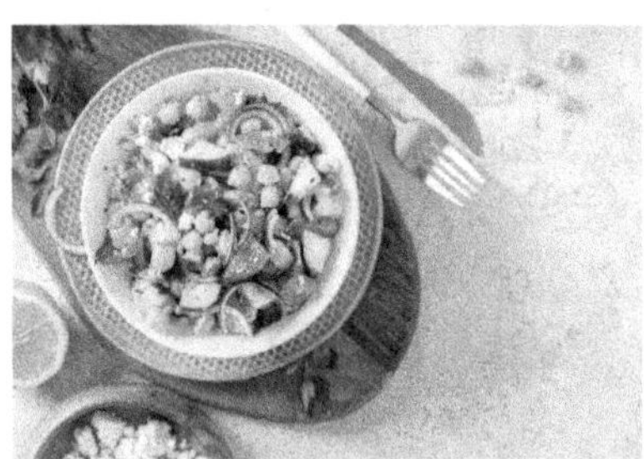

Meditterenean Chicpea salad with tomato, cucumber, feta cheese, parsley, onions and lemon

o **Quinoa and Spinach Salad**: Mix cooked quinoa with baby spinach, sliced almonds, dried cranberries, and crumbled goat cheese. Top with a balsamic vinaigrette.

o **Tabbouleh Salad**: Combine chopped fresh parsley, diced tomatoes, diced cucumber, finely chopped red onion, cooked bulgur, and a generous squeeze of lemon juice. Drizzle with olive oil.

o **Caprese Salad**: Arrange slices of ripe tomatoes, fresh mozzarella, and basil leaves on a plate. Drizzle with balsamic glaze and extra virgin olive oil. Season with salt and pepper.

o **Mediterranean Orzo Salad**: Toss cooked orzo pasta with diced cucumber, cherry tomatoes, red onion, chopped Kalamata olives, crumbled feta, and a lemon-herb dressing.

- **Lemon-Oregano Vinaigrette**: Whisk together 1/4 cup of extra virgin olive oil, 2 tablespoons of lemon juice, 1 teaspoon of dried oregano, 1 minced garlic clove, salt, and pepper.

- **Balsamic Vinaigrette**: Mix 1/4 cup of balsamic vinegar, 1/4 cup of extra virgin olive oil, 1 teaspoon of Dijon mustard, 1 minced garlic clove, and a touch of honey. Season with salt and pepper.

- **Tahini Yogurt Dressing**: In a bowl, combine 1/4 cup of tahini, 1/4 cup of plain Greek yogurt, 2 tablespoons of lemon juice, 1 minced garlic clove, and water to reach the desired consistency. Season with salt and pepper.

- **Mint-Dill Dressing**: Blend together a handful of fresh mint leaves, a handful of fresh dill, 1/4 cup of Greek yogurt, 2 tablespoons of white wine vinegar, and 1 tablespoon of honey. Thin with water if needed.

- **Basil-Lemon Dressing**: In a blender, combine 1 cup of fresh basil leaves, 1/4 cup of extra virgin olive oil, 2 tablespoons of lemon juice, 1 minced garlic clove, salt, and pepper.

These salad ideas and dressing recipes highlight the vibrant flavors of the Mediterranean region. They're perfect for enjoying as a light and nutritious meal or as a refreshing side dish for any occasion.

5.1 Nourishing salads with PCOS-friendly ingredients

Here are some nourishing Mediterranean-inspired salads featuring PCOS-friendly ingredients that are rich in nutrients and support blood sugar regulation:

i. Mediterranean Quinoa Salad:

- Mix cooked quinoa with chopped cucumbers, bell peppers, cherry tomatoes, red onion, and chopped fresh parsley.
- Add Kalamata olives, crumbled feta cheese, and a handful of chickpeas for protein.
- Drizzle with a lemon-oregano vinaigrette made with extra virgin olive oil, lemon juice, dried oregano, garlic, salt, and pepper.

ii. Spinach and Berry Salad:

- o Combine baby spinach with a mix of berries (blueberries, strawberries and raspberries).
- o Top with chopped walnuts, crumbled goat cheese, and grilled chicken or turkey.
- o Drizzle with a balsamic vinaigrette made with extra virgin olive oil, balsamic vinegar, Dijon mustard, minced garlic, and a touch of honey.

iii. Greek Lentil Salad:

- o Toss cooked green or brown lentils with diced cucumber, red bell pepper, red onion, cherry tomatoes, and chopped fresh mint.
- o Add crumbled feta cheese and a handful of chopped almonds for crunch.
- o Drizzle with a lemon-tahini dressing made with tahini, lemon juice, minced garlic, water, salt, and pepper.i

iv. Roasted Vegetable and Chickpea Salad:

- o Roast a mix of colorful vegetables like sweet potatoes, bell peppers, zucchini, and red onions with olive oil, garlic, and dried herbs.

- o Toss the roasted veggies with cooked chickpeas and a bed of mixed greens.
- o Top with a light dressing made from extra virgin olive oil, lemon juice, a touch of honey, and chopped fresh thyme.

v. Greek Salad with Avocado:

- o Combine chopped cucumbers, tomatoes, red onion, Kalamata olives, and crumbled feta cheese with mixed greens.
- o Add diced avocado for healthy fats and creaminess.
- o Drizzle with a simple dressing made from extra virgin olive oil, lemon juice, dried oregano, salt, and pepper.

These salads incorporate a variety of colorful vegetables, lean proteins, healthy fats, and whole grains, making them ideal for individuals with PCOS. The Mediterranean-inspired flavors and nutrient-rich ingredients make these salads satisfying and nourishing choices.

5.2 Homemade dressings to elevate your salad game

Elevate your salad game with these homemade dressings that add flavor and nutrition to your Mediterranean-inspired salads:

- o **Lemon-Tahini Dressing**: Whisk together 1/4 cup tahini, 2 tablespoons lemon juice, 1 clove minced garlic, 2 tablespoons water, a pinch of cumin, salt, and pepper. Adjust the water for the desired consistency.

- o **Greek Yogurt Cucumber Dill Dressing**: Blend 1/2 cup plain Greek yogurt, 1/4 cup diced cucumber, 2 tablespoons chopped fresh dill, 1 tablespoon lemon juice, 1 clove minced garlic, salt, and pepper.

- o **Balsamic-Orange Vinaigrette**: Mix 1/4 cup balsamic vinegar, 2 tablespoons freshly squeezed orange juice, 1 teaspoon Dijon mustard, 1 teaspoon honey, 1/2 cup extra virgin olive oil, salt, and pepper.

- o **Mint-Basil Pesto Dressing**:In a blender, combine 1 cup fresh basil leaves, 1/2 cup fresh

mint leaves, 1/4 cup pine nuts, 1/4 cup grated
Parmesan cheese, 1 clove garlic, 1/2 cup extra
virgin olive oil, salt, and pepper.

o **Lemon-Honey Olive Oil Dressing**: Whisk
together 1/4 cup extra virgin olive oil, 2
tablespoons lemon juice, 1 tablespoon honey, 1
teaspoon Dijon mustard, minced garlic, salt, and
pepper.

o **Greek Feta Dressing**: Mash 1/4 cup crumbled
feta cheese with 2 tablespoons plain Greek
yogurt, 2 tablespoons lemon juice, 1 clove
minced garlic, dried oregano, salt, and pepper.

o **Mediterranean Herb Dressing**: Combine 1/4
cup extra virgin olive oil, 2 tablespoons red wine
vinegar, 1 teaspoon dried oregano, 1/2 teaspoon
dried thyme, minced garlic, salt, and pepper.

o **Basil-Lemon Vinaigrette**: Blend 1 cup fresh
basil leaves, 1/4 cup extra virgin olive oil, 2
tablespoons lemon juice, 1 teaspoon Dijon
mustard, 1 clove minced garlic, salt, and pepper.

- o **Creamy Avocado-Lime Dressing**: Blend together 1 ripe avocado, 1/4 cup plain Greek yogurt, 2 tablespoons lime juice, 1 clove minced garlic, a handful of fresh cilantro, water to thin, salt, and pepper.

- o **Orange-Mint Dressing**: Mix 1/4 cup freshly squeezed orange juice, 2 tablespoons extra virgin olive oil, 1 tablespoon chopped fresh mint, 1 teaspoon honey, a pinch of ground cumin, salt, and pepper.

These homemade dressings can be a game-changer, adding depth and complexity to your salads while keeping them wholesome and nutrient-rich. Customize the flavors to your liking and enjoy the burst of Mediterranean-inspired tastes on your plate

Chapter 6: Satisfying Soups And Stews

Here are some satisfying Mediterranean-inspired soup and stew ideas that are not only delicious but also packed with wholesome ingredients:

a. Lentil and Vegetable Stew:

- o Sauté onions, carrots, and celery in olive oil until softened. Add red lentils, diced tomatoes, vegetable broth, and a mix of Mediterranean herbs (like thyme, rosemary, and oregano).
- o Simmer until the lentils are tender. Add chopped spinach or kale towards the end. Season with salt and pepper.

b. Mediterranean Fish Stew:

- o In a pot, sauté garlic, onions, and bell peppers in olive oil. Add canned diced tomatoes, vegetable or fish broth, and a pinch of saffron for flavor.
- o Gently place pieces of white fish (like cod or haddock) into the broth and cook until the fish is cooked through. Add a handful of chopped fresh parsley before serving.

c. Chickpea and Spinach Soup:

- o Cook chickpeas until tender (canned or soaked and boiled). In a pot, sauté chopped onions, garlic, and carrots in olive oil.
- o Add cooked chickpeas, vegetable broth, and chopped spinach. Season with cumin, paprika, and a squeeze of lemon juice.

d. Tomato and Vegetable Soup:

- o Sauté onions, carrots, celery, and bell peppers in olive oil. Add canned tomato puree, vegetable broth, and chopped zucchini.
- o Simmer until the vegetables are tender. Season with Italian herbs like basil, oregano, and thyme. Add cooked whole- wheat pasta for extra heartiness.

e. Mediterranean Bean Stew:

- o Sauté chopped onions, garlic, and bell peppers in olive oil. Add canned mixed beans (like cannellini, kidney, and black beans), diced tomatoes, and vegetable broth.
- o Stir in chopped kale or Swiss chard and let it wilt. Season with dried herbs like rosemary and thyme.

f. Roasted Vegetable Soup:

- o Roast a variety of Mediterranean vegetables (eggplant, zucchini, bell peppers and tomatoes) with olive oil and garlic until caramelized.
- o Blend the roasted vegetables with the vegetable broth until smooth. Season with basil, oregano, and a touch of balsamic vinegar.

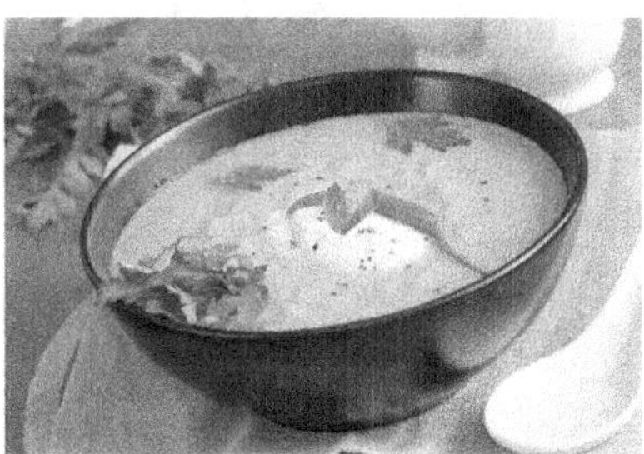

Roasted Squash and Chili soup

g. Greek Lemon Chicken Soup (Avgolemono):

- o Simmer chicken broth with cooked shredded chicken, orzo pasta, and diced carrots until the pasta is cooked.
- o In a separate bowl, whisk together the eggs and lemon juice. Gradually temper the egg mixture with a ladle of hot broth.

o   Slowly add the tempered egg mixture back to the soup, stirring constantly until the soup thickens. Season with dill and salt.

h. Mediterranean Minestrone:

o   In a pot, sauté onions, garlic, carrots, and celery in olive oil. Add vegetable broth, canned diced tomatoes, cooked small pasta, and a mix of Mediterranean vegetables like green beans and zucchini.

o   Simmer until the vegetables are tender. Season with Italian herbs and garnish with grated Parmesan.

These Mediterranean-inspired soup and stew ideas are not only comforting but also filled with a variety of vegetables, legumes, and lean proteins. They offer a balance of flavors and nutrients, making them ideal for nourishing meals

6.1 Hearty soups and stews infused with Mediterranean flavors

Here are some hearty Mediterranean-inspired soups and stews that bring together rich flavors and wholesome ingredients:

i. Mediterranean Vegetable Stew:

- o Sauté onions, garlic, and bell peppers in olive oil. Add diced eggplant, zucchini, and canned tomatoes.
- o Season with a mix of Mediterranean herbs like oregano, thyme, and rosemary.
- o Add cooked chickpeas and vegetable broth. Simmer until vegetables are tender. Garnish with chopped fresh parsley.

ii. Seafood and Fennel Stew:

- o Sauté chopped fennel, onions, and garlic in olive oil. Add diced tomatoes, fish or seafood broth, and a touch of white wine.
- o Gently add pieces of your choice of seafood (like shrimp, mussels, and fish).
- o Season with saffron, dried basil, and a squeeze of lemon juice. Simmer until the seafood is cooked.

iii. Lamb and White Bean Stew:

- o Brown cubed lamb meat in a pot with olive oil. Remove and set aside.
- o Sauté onions, carrots, and celery. Add diced tomatoes, cooked white beans, and lamb back into the pot.

- o Add lamb or beef broth, a splash of red wine, and a blend of Mediterranean spices like cumin, coriander, and paprika.
- o Simmer until the meat is tender. Garnish with chopped fresh mint.

iv. Spiced Lentil and Tomato Soup:

- o Sauté onions, garlic, and carrots in olive oil. Add dried red lentils, canned diced tomatoes, and vegetable broth.
- o Season with cumin smoked paprika, and a pinch of cinnamon.
- o Simmer until the lentils are cooked. Add chopped Swiss chard or spinach before serving.

v. Chicken and Olive Stew:

- o Sear chicken pieces in olive oil until golden. Remove and set aside.
- o Sauté onions, garlic, and bell peppers. Add diced tomatoes, chicken broth, and chicken back to the pot.
- o Add pitted Kalamata olives, dried oregano, and a splash of red wine vinegar.
- o Simmer until the chicken is cooked through. Garnish with chopped fresh basil.

vi. Mushroom and Barley Soup:

- o Sauté sliced mushrooms and chopped onions in
    olive oil until browned.
- o Add the pearl barley, vegetable broth, and diced
    tomatoes.
- o Season with rosemary, thyme, and a splash of
    balsamic vinegar.
- o Simmer until the barley is tender. Top with
    grated Parmesan.

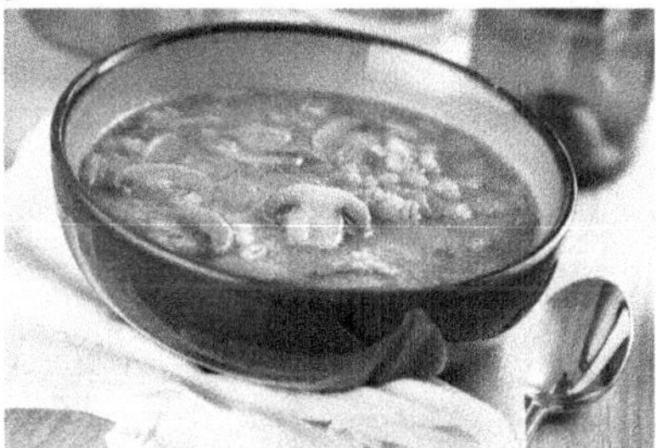

**A bowl of homemade mushroom and barley
soup**

v. Lentil and Sausage Stew:

- o Brown the Italian sausage in a pot. Remove and
    set aside.
- o Sauté onions, carrots, and celery. Add dried
    brown lentils, diced tomatoes, and chicken or
    vegetable broth.
- o Season with Italian herbs like basil, oregano, and
    thyme.

o   Simmer until the lentils are cooked. Stir in sliced cooked sausage before serving.

vi. Harira Soup (Moroccan Lentil Soup):

o   Sauté onions, celery, and bell peppers in olive oil. Add dried red lentils and diced tomatoes.
o   Season with Moroccan spices like cumin, coriander, and cinnamon.
o   Add vegetable broth and chopped fresh cilantro and parsley.
o   Simmer until the lentils are tender. Serve with a squeeze of lemon.

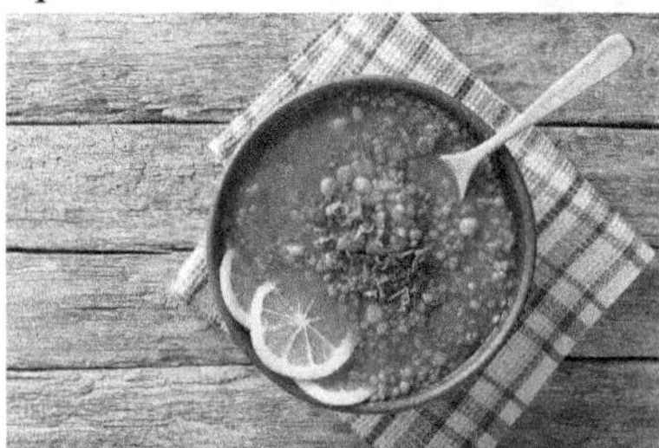

A bowl of Harira soup

These hearty soups and stews are infused with Mediterranean flavors, using ingredients that create a warm and satisfying meal while incorporating the healthful essence of the Mediterranean Diet.

6.2 Rich and comforting meals for a nourishing experience

Here are some rich and comforting Mediterranean-inspired meal ideas that provide a nourishing experience:

i. Eggplant Parmesan:

- Layer slices of roasted or breaded and baked eggplant with marinara sauce and mozzarella cheese.
- Bake until the cheese is melted and bubbly. Serve over whole wheat pasta or with a side salad.

ii. Mediterranean Baked Chicken:

- Marinate chicken breasts with olive oil, lemon juice, minced garlic, dried oregano, and a touch of paprika.
- Bake until cooked through, and serve with a side of roasted vegetables and quinoa.

iii. Lamb and Eggplant Moussaka:

- Layer sautéed ground lamb, roasted eggplant, and a creamy béchamel sauce in a baking dish.
- Bake until golden and serve as a hearty casserole.

iv. Stuffed Bell Peppers:

- o Fill bell pepper halves with a mixture of cooked ground turkey, quinoa, chopped tomatoes, diced zucchini, and spices.
- o Top with feta cheese and bake until the the peppers are tender.

v. Chicken Shawarma Wraps:

- o Marinate chicken in a blend of yogurt, lemon juice, garlic, cumin, paprika, and turmeric.
- o Grill or sauté the chicken and serve in whole wheat wraps with a Greek yogurt tzatziki sauce and fresh veggies.

vi. Lentil and Sausage Casserole:

- o Sauté Italian sausage and set aside. In the same pot, sauté onions, carrots, and celery.
- o Add dried lentils, diced tomatoes, and vegetable broth. Season with Italian herbs.
- o Stir in the cooked sausage and simmer until the lentils are tender.

v. Mediterranean Pasta Primavera:

- o Toss whole wheat pasta with a variety of sautéed Mediterranean vegetables like zucchini, bell peppers, cherry tomatoes, and spinach.
- o Drizzle with olive oil, lemon zest, and grated Parmesan.

vi. Beef and Vegetable Stew:

- o Sear beef cubes and set aside. Sauté onions, garlic, and carrots in olive oil.
- o Add the beef back to the pot along with diced tomatoes, beef broth, and a mix of Mediterranean herbs.
- o Simmer until the beef is tender. Serve with crusty whole-grain bread.

vii. Greek Spinach and Feta Pie (Spanakopita):

- o Layer the spinach and feta mixture between sheets of phyllo dough. Bake until golden and crisp.
- o Serve as individual triangles or as a larger pie.

viii. Mediterranean Stuffed Acorn Squash:

- o Roast halved acorn squash. Fill with a mixture of cooked quinoa, chickpeas, diced tomatoes, and chopped fresh herbs.
- o Top with crumbled feta and bake until heated through.

These nourishing and comforting Mediterranean-inspired meals bring together a variety of flavors, textures, and nutrients to create satisfying dishes that are perfect for enjoying with family and friends.

Chapter 7: Seafood Specialties

Here are some delicious Mediterranean-inspired seafood specialties that showcase the flavors of the sea and the Mediterranean region:

i. Grilled Mediterranean Fish:

- o Marinate fish fillets (like sea bass, red snapper, or salmon) with olive oil, lemon juice, minced garlic, and a mix of fresh herbs such as thyme, rosemary, and oregano.
- o Grill the fish until cooked through, and serve with a side of roasted vegetables or a salad.

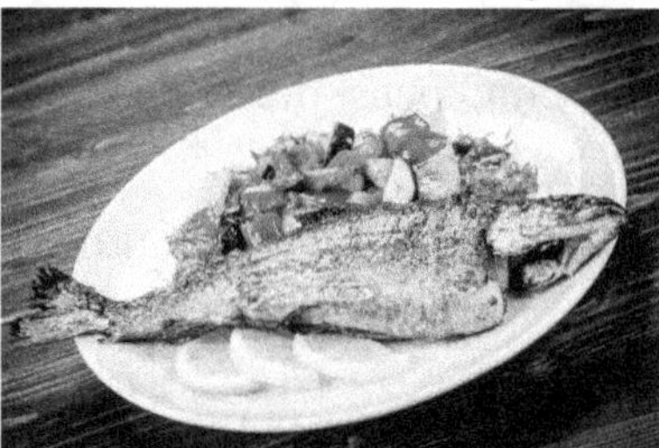

Grilled Mediterranean fish with roasted vegetable

ii. Mediterranean Seafood Paella:

- o Sauté onions, bell peppers, and garlic in olive oil. Add Arborio rice and cook until lightly toasted.
- o Add saffron, diced tomatoes, fish broth, and a mix of seafood (shrimp, mussels and squid).
- o Simmer until the rice is cooked and the seafood is tender. Garnish with chopped parsley.

iii. Baked Stuffed Fish:

- o Fill whole fish (like branzino or trout) with a mixture of breadcrumbs, chopped fresh herbs, garlic, lemon zest, and olive oil.
- o Bake the fish until the flesh flakes easily. Serve with a squeeze of lemon.

iv. Sicilian-Style Grilled Swordfish:

- o Marinate swordfish steaks in olive oil, lemon juice, minced garlic, and chopped fresh mint.
- o Grill the swordfish until charred and cooked through. Serve with a caper and olive relish.

v. Greek-style Shrimp Saganaki:

- o Sauté shrimp with onions, garlic, and diced tomatoes in a skillet. Add white wine, crumbled feta, and chopped fresh parsley.
- o Simmer until the shrimp are cooked and the feta is melted. Serve with crusty bread.

vi. Mediterranean Ceviche:

- o Marinate diced white fish (like sea bass or halibut) in freshly squeezed lemon and lime juice.
- o Add diced tomatoes, red onion, cucumber, bell peppers, and chopped cilantro.
- o Serve the ceviche chilled with pita chips.

vii. Mussel and Tomato Stew:

- o Sauté onions, garlic, and diced tomatoes in olive oil. Add cleaned mussels and white wine.
- o Cover and simmer until the mussels open. Serve with crusty bread for dipping.

viii. Grilled Octopus Salad:

- o Tenderize the octopus by boiling it, and then marinate it with olive oil, lemon juice, oregano, and garlic.
- o Grill the octopus until charred and serve it on a bed of mixed greens with olives and roasted red peppers.

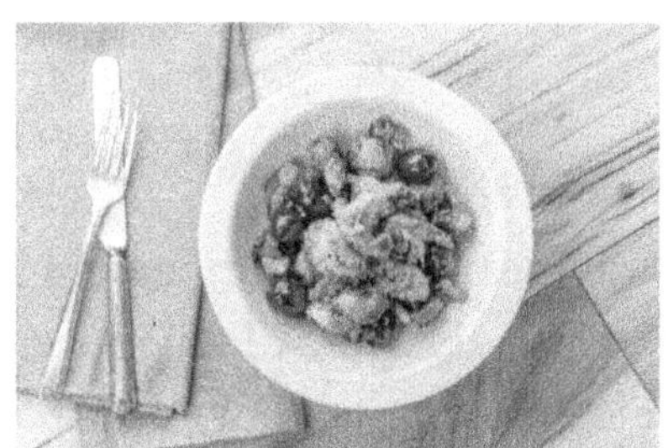

Octopus salad

ix. Lemon-Herb Baked Salmon:

- o Coat salmon fillets with a mixture of lemon zest, chopped fresh dill, minced garlic, and olive oil.
- o Bake the salmon until it flakes easily. Serve with a side of steamed vegetables or quinoa.

x. Italian-Style Calamari:

- o Sauté calamari rings with garlic, cherry tomatoes, and red pepper flakes in olive oil.
- o Add white wine and a squeeze of lemon juice. Serve over pasta or with crusty bread.

These Mediterranean seafood specialties showcase the diverse and flavorful ways that seafood can be prepared to capture the essence of the Mediterranean diet. Enjoy the wonderful tastes of the sea with these dishes!

7.1 Seafood recipes rich in Omega-3s for PCOS support

Including omega-3-rich seafood in your diet can be beneficial for PCOS. Here are some Mediterranean-inspired seafood recipes that are not only delicious but also provide a good source of omega-3 fatty acids:

i. Salmon and Quinoa Bowl:

- Grill or bake salmon fillets seasoned with olive oil, lemon juice, and a sprinkle of dried dill.
- Serve the salmon over cooked quinoa and a bed of mixed greens.
- Top with diced cucumber, cherry tomatoes, red onion, and a drizzle of tahini dressing.

ii. Mediterranean Tuna Salad:

- Mix canned tuna (packed in water) with diced cucumber, Kalamata olives, chopped red onion, and chopped fresh parsley.
- Toss with extra virgin olive oil, lemon juice, dried oregano, and a pinch of crushed red pepper.
- Serve the tuna salad over a bed of baby spinach or arugula.

iii. Omega-3 -Packed Sardine Toast:

- o Mash canned sardines (packed in olive oil) with chopped fresh herbs, lemon zest, and a touch of Dijon mustard.
- o Spread the sardine mixture on whole- grain toast and top with sliced radishes and arugula.

iv. Grilled Mackerel with Citrus Salsa:

- o Marinate mackerel fillets with olive oil, minced garlic, lemon zest, and chopped fresh thyme.
- o Grill the mackerel until it's cooked through and slightly crispy.
- o Serve with a salsa made from diced oranges, grapefruit, red onion, and chopped mint.

v. Herb-Roasted Trout:

- o Coat trout fillets with a mixture of chopped fresh rosemary, thyme, and parsley mixed with olive oil and lemon juice.
- o Roast the trout in the oven until it's tender and flakes easily.
- o Serve with a side of steamed broccoli and quinoa.

vi. Greek-Style Anchovy and Olive Pasta:

- o Sauté diced anchovies (packed in olive oil) with chopped garlic, black olives, and cherry tomatoes in olive oil.

- o Toss with whole wheat pasta and a handful of baby spinach.
- o Finish with a sprinkle of grated Parmesan.

vii. Walnut-Crusted Cod:

- o Coat cod fillets with a mixture of crushed walnuts, whole wheat breadcrumbs, and dried thyme.
- o Bake the cod until it's cooked and the crust is golden.
- o Serve with a side of roasted sweet potatoes and a green salad.

viii. Lemon-Herb Chia Seed Crusted Tilapia:

- o Coat tilapia fillets with a mixture of chia seeds, lemon zest, chopped fresh herbs, and olive oil.
- o Pan-fry the tilapia until it's crispy and cooked through.
- o Serve with a side of quinoa and sautéed spinach.

These omega-3-rich seafood recipes incorporate flavorful Mediterranean ingredients and offer a variety of options for incorporating the benefits of omega-3 fatty acids into your diet while supporting PCOS management.

7.2 Grilled, baked, and pan-seared delicacies

Here are some grilled, baked, and pan-seared Mediterranean delicacies that offer a variety of flavors and cooking techniques:

i. Grilled Lemon-Herb Shrimp Skewers:

- o Marinate shrimp in olive oil, lemon juice, minced garlic, chopped fresh herbs (like rosemary and thyme), and a pinch of red pepper flakes.
- o Thread the shrimp onto skewers and grill until they're pink and slightly charred.

ii. Baked Stuffed Clams:

- o Mix chopped clams with breadcrumbs, minced garlic, chopped fresh parsley, and grated Parmesan.
- o Stuff the mixture back into the clam shells and bake until golden and crispy.

iii. Pan-Seared Scallops with Mango Salsa:

- o Season scallops with salt, pepper, and a touch of paprika. Pan-sear them until they're caramelized on both sides.
- o Serve with a fresh salsa made from diced mango, red onion, cilantro, and lime juice.

iii. Grilled Swordfish Steak with Olive Tapenade:

- o Grill swordfish steaks and serve them topped with a flavorful olive tapenade made from Kalamata olives, capers, chopped fresh herbs, and olive oil.

iv. Baked Stuffed Lobster Tails:

- o Split lobster tails in half lengthwise and stuff with a mixture of breadcrumbs, butter, minced garlic, chopped fresh parsley, and lemon zest.
- o Bake until the lobster is cooked and the stuffing is golden.

v. Pan-Seared Calamari Steaks:

- o Season calamari steaks with salt, pepper, and a sprinkle of smoked paprika.
- o Sear them in a hot pan until they're charred and cooked through.

vi. Grilled Whole Branzino:

- o Marinate whole branzino (European seabass) with olive oil, lemon slices, chopped fresh herbs, and garlic.
- o Grill the branzino until the skin is crispy and the flesh is flaky.

vii. Baked Mussels with Herbed Breadcrumbs:

- o   Top cleaned mussels with a mixture of breadcrumbs, chopped fresh herbs, lemon zest, and a drizzle of olive oil.
- o   Bake until the breadcrumbs are golden and the mussels have opened.

viii. Pan-Seared Red Snapper with Tomato-Caper Relish:

- o   Pan-sear red snapper fillets until they're crispy on the outside and tender on the inside.
- o   Serve with a relish made from diced tomatoes, capers, red onion, and balsamic vinegar.

ix. Grilled Octopus with Lemon-Garlic Marinade:

- o   Tenderize the octopus by boiling it, charring it, and then marinate it in a mixture of olive oil, lemon juice, minced garlic, and fresh oregano.
- o   Grill the octopus until it's charred, and serve with a squeeze of lemon.

These grilled, baked, and pan-seared delicacies capture the essence of Mediterranean cuisine, focusing on fresh ingredients and a variety of cooking methods that enhance the flavors of the seafood.

Chapter 8: Poultry and Lean Meats

Here are some Mediterranean-inspired recipes featuring poultry and lean meats that highlight the region's flavors and wholesome ingredients:

i. Lemon-Herb Grilled Chicken:

- o Marinate chicken breasts in a mixture of olive oil, lemon juice, minced garlic, chopped fresh herbs (like oregano and thyme), and a touch of paprika.
- o Grill the chicken until it's cooked through, and serve with a side of Greek salad.

ii. Mediterranean Turkey Meatballs:

- o Mix ground turkey with chopped fresh parsley, minced garlic, diced red onion, and a blend of Mediterranean spices (cumin, coriander and paprika).
- o Form into meatballs and bake in the oven. Serve with a yogurt-based tzatziki sauce.

iii. Balsamic-Glazed Chicken Thighs:

- o Coat chicken thighs with a balsamic glaze made from balsamic vinegar, honey, minced garlic, and dried Italian herbs.
- o Bake the chicken until it's caramelized, and serve with roasted vegetables.

iv. Greek-Style Yogurt Marinated Lamb Chops:

- o Marinate lamb chops in a mixture of Greek yogurt, lemon juice, minced garlic, chopped fresh mint, and rosemary.
- o Grill the lamb chops until they're cooked to your desired level of doneness.

v. Pan-Seared Lemon-Herb Turkey Cutlets:

- o Season turkey cutlets with salt, pepper, and a mixture of chopped fresh herbs (such as rosemary and thyme).
- o Pan-sear the cutlets until they're golden and cooked through. Serve with a squeeze of lemon.

vi. Herb-Crusted Pork Tenderloin:

- o Coat pork tenderloin with a mixture of whole wheat breadcrumbs, chopped fresh herbs, lemon zest, and olive oil.
- o Roast the pork in the oven until it's tender and the crust is golden.

vii. Mediterranean Chicken Skewers:

- o Thread chunks of chicken breast onto skewers and marinate in olive oil, lemon juice, minced garlic, dried oregano, and red pepper flakes.
- o Grill the skewers until the chicken is cooked and slightly charred. Serve with pita bread and tzatziki.

viii. Italian-Style Grilled Steak:

- o Marinate lean steak (like sirloin) in olive oil, balsamic vinegar, minced garlic, dried basil, and oregano.

- o Grill the steak to your preferred doneness and serve with a side of roasted vegetables.

ix. Roasted Herb-Crusted Chicken:

- o Rub chicken with a mixture of chopped fresh herbs, minced garlic, lemon zest, and olive oil.
- o Roast the chicken until it's golden and cooked through. Serve with whole grains and steamed greens.

x. Lemon-Rosemary Grilled Turkey Breast:

- o Marinate turkey breast in a blend of olive oil, lemon juice, chopped fresh rosemary, and a touch of Dijon mustard.
- o Grill the turkey until it's juicy and cooked. Serve with a side of quinoa and grilled vegetables.

These Mediterranean-inspired poultry and lean meat recipes combine lean protein sources with flavorful herbs and spices, delivering a delightful and nutritious culinary experience.

8.1 Protein-packed dishes using lean meats and poultry

Here are some protein-packed Mediterranean-inspired dishes using lean meats and poultry:

i. Greek Chicken Souvlaki:

- o Marinate chicken breast cubes in olive oil, lemon juice, minced garlic, dried oregano, and a touch of red pepper flakes.
- o Thread onto skewers and grill until cooked through. Serve with whole wheat pita, Greek salad, and tzatziki.

ii. Mediterranean Turkey and Spinach Stuffed Bell Peppers:

- o Mix ground turkey with chopped spinach, cooked quinoa, diced tomatoes, minced garlic, and Mediterranean spices.
- o Stuff the mixture into bell peppers and bake until the peppers are tender and filling is cooked.

iii. Grilled Lemon-Herb Pork Tenderloin:

- o Marinate pork tenderloin in a mixture of olive oil, lemon zest, minced garlic, chopped fresh rosemary, and thyme.
- o Grill the pork until cooked, and serve with a side of grilled vegetables.

iv. Chicken and Chickpea Stew:

o   Sauté diced chicken breast with onions, bell peppers, and minced garlic in olive oil.
o   Add canned chickpeas, diced tomatoes, chicken broth, and a blend of Mediterranean spices. Simmer until flavors meld.

v. Mediterranean Beef Kebabs:

o   Marinate lean beef chunks in olive oil, red wine vinegar, minced garlic, dried oregano, and paprika.
o   Skewer the beef with bell peppers, onions, and tomatoes. Grill until beef is done. Serve with couscous.

vi. Lemon-Rosemary Grilled Chicken Salad:

o   Grill marinated chicken breasts and slice them.
o   Arrange sliced chicken on a bed of mixed greens with cherry tomatoes, cucumber, olives, and feta cheese.
o   Drizzle with a lemon-rosemary vinaigrette.

vii. Turkey and Vegetable Stir-Fry:

o   Sauté sliced turkey breast with a mix of colorful vegetables (like bell peppers, zucchini, and snap peas) in a stir-fry sauce made from low-sodium soy sauce, ginger, and garlic.

viii. Mediterranean Lean Beef Meatball Bowl:

- o Make lean beef meatballs seasoned with chopped fresh herbs and spices. Bake until cooked.
- o Serve the meatballs over a bowl of quinoa or brown rice with roasted vegetables and hummus.

ix. Lemon-Dijon Grilled Chicken Wrap:

- o Grill chicken breast marinated in lemon juice, Dijon mustard, minced garlic, and thyme.
- o Wrap the grilled chicken in a whole wheat tortilla with mixed greens, diced tomatoes, and a dollop of Greek yogurt.

x. Greek-Style Ground Turkey Skillet:

- o Sauté ground turkey with onions, bell peppers, and diced tomatoes in olive oil.
- o Add Mediterranean spices like oregano, thyme, and cumin. Serve over couscous or whole wheat pasta.

These protein-packed dishes combine lean meats and poultry with a variety of Mediterranean-inspired ingredients and flavors, offering both deliciousness and nutritional value.

8.2 Balanced meals for a PCOS-friendly diet

Creating balanced meals is essential for a PCOS-friendly diet. Here are some Mediterranean-inspired balanced meal ideas that incorporate a variety of nutrients to support PCOS management:

1. Breakfast:

Mediterranean Omelette:

- Make an omelette with egg whites or a mix of whole eggs and egg whites.
- Fill it with sautéed spinach, diced tomatoes, bell peppers, and a sprinkle of feta cheese.
- Serve with a slice of whole grain toast and a side of fresh fruit.

2. Lunch:

Quinoa and Chickpea Salad

- Toss cooked quinoa with canned chickpeas, diced cucumbers, cherry tomatoes, chopped fresh parsley, and red onion.
- Drizzle with a lemon-herb vinaigrette made from olive oil, lemon juice, minced garlic, and dried oregano.

    o Top with grilled chicken or canned tuna for added protein.

3.. Snack:

Greek Yogurt Parfait.

    o Layer plain Greek yogurt with mixed berries, a drizzle of honey, and a sprinkle of chopped nuts (like almonds or walnuts).

4. Dinner:

Baked Salmon with Roasted Vegetables.

    o Bake salmon fillets seasoned with olive oil, lemon juice, minced garlic, and dill.
    o Serve the salmon with a side of roasted Mediterranean vegetables (eggplant, zucchini, and bell peppers) and a small serving of whole grain (like quinoa or farro).

5.Snack:

Veggie Sticks with Hummus

    o Enjoy carrot, cucumber, and bell pepper sticks with a portion of hummus for dipping.

Remember to focus on whole, nutrient-dense foods and include a balance of lean proteins, complex carbohydrates, healthy fats, and plenty of colorful vegetables. The Mediterranean diet's emphasis on fresh produce, lean proteins, and healthy fats can provide a solid foundation for a PCOS-friendly eating plan.

Chapter 9: Abundant Vegetarian Entrees

Here are some abundant vegetarian entree ideas that are rich in nutrients and flavors:

i. Mediterranean Chickpea Stew:

- o Sauté onions, bell peppers, and zucchini in olive oil. Add canned chickpeas, diced tomatoes, vegetable broth, and a mix of Mediterranean herbs.

- o Simmer until vegetables are tender. Serve with whole wheat couscous or crusty bread.

ii. Eggplant Parmesan Stack:

- o Layer slices of breaded and baked eggplant with marinara sauce and slices of fresh mozzarella.
- o Bake until the cheese is melted and bubbly. Serve with a side salad.

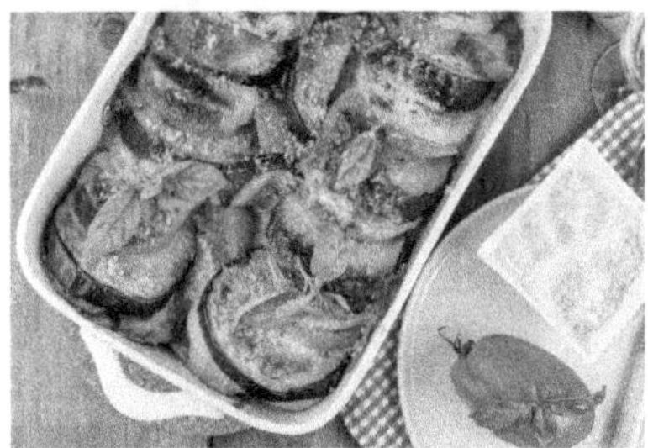

iii. Mushroom and Spinach Stuffed Peppers:

- o Sauté mushrooms, spinach, onions, and garlic in olive oil. Mix with cooked quinoa and crumbled feta.
- o Stuff bell peppers with the mixture and bake until the peppers are tender.

iv. Mediterranean Lentil Salad:

- o Toss cooked green lentils with diced cucumbers, cherry tomatoes, red onion, Kalamata olives, and chopped fresh parsley.

o   Drizzle with a lemon-herb vinaigrette and crumbled feta cheese.

v. Greek-style Stuffed Tomatoes:

o   Hollow out large tomatoes and fill them with a mixture of cooked bulgur, diced cucumber, red onion, chopped fresh mint, and lemon juice.
o   Top with crumbled feta and bake until tomatoes are heated.

vi. Mediterranean Grilled Veggie Wrap:

o   Grill eggplant, zucchini, and bell peppers. Wrap the grilled vegetables in a whole wheat tortilla with hummus and a sprinkle of crumbled goat cheese.

vii. Spinach and Feta Stuffed Portobello Mushrooms:

o   Sauté spinach, garlic, and diced tomatoes in olive oil. Mix with crumbled feta.

- o Stuff portobello mushroom caps with the mixture
    and bake until the mushrooms are tender.

viii. Greek Pasta Salad:

- o Toss cooked whole wheat pasta with diced
    cucumbers, cherry tomatoes, red onion, Kalamata
    olives, crumbled feta, and chopped fresh parsley.
- o Drizzle with olive oil and lemon dressing.

ix. Mediterranean Quinoa Bowl:

- o Build a bowl with cooked quinoa, roasted
    chickpeas, grilled artichoke hearts, sliced
    avocado, diced cucumber, and a dollop of
    tzatziki.

x. Spanakopita (Spinach Pie):

- o Layer phyllo dough with a mixture of sautéed
    spinach, onions, garlic, feta cheese, and chopped
    fresh dill.
- o Bake until the phyllo is golden and crispy.

These abundant vegetarian entrees celebrate the flavors
of the Mediterranean with a variety of vegetables,

legumes, and whole grains, offering a satisfying and nourishing dining experience.

9.1 Vibrant and diverse plant-based dishes for every palate

Here's a selection of vibrant and diverse plant-based dishes inspired by Mediterranean flavors that cater to various palates:

i. Stuffed Bell Peppers with Quinoa and Black Beans:

- o Mix cooked quinoa with black beans, corn, diced tomatoes, and chopped cilantro.
- o Stuff bell peppers with the mixture and bake until the peppers are tender.

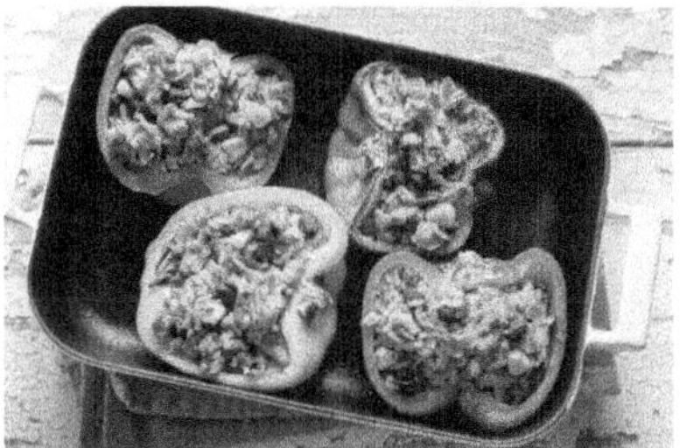

Stuffed bell peppers with black beans

ii. Mediterranean Veggie Burger:

- o Create a patty with a blend of cooked quinoa, chickpeas, diced olives, chopped sun-dried tomatoes, and Mediterranean spices.
- o Serve the patty on a whole-grain bun with lettuce, tomato, and a dollop of hummus.

iii. Zucchini Noodles with Pesto and Cherry Tomatoes:

- o Spiralize zucchini into noodles and toss with homemade basil pesto and halved cherry tomatoes.
- o Top with toasted pine nuts and a sprinkle of nutritional yeast.

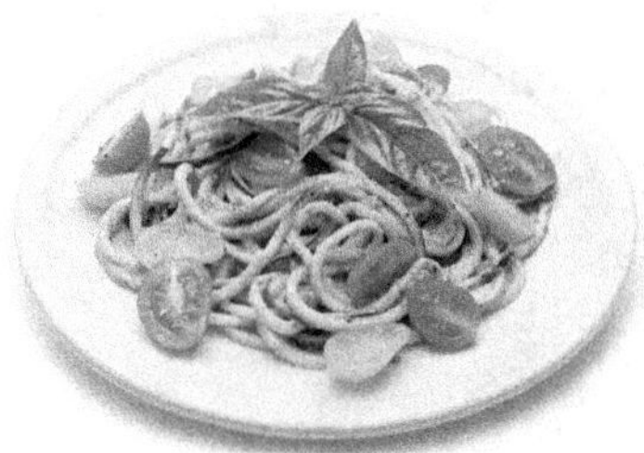

iv. Cauliflower and Chickpea Shawarma Bowl:

- o Roast cauliflower and chickpeas with shawarma spices until they're crispy.
- o Serve over a bed of mixed greens with diced cucumbers, red onion, and a tahini drizzle.

v. Greek-style Lentil Salad:

- o Toss cooked green lentils with diced cucumbers, cherry tomatoes, red onion, Kalamata olives, and crumbled vegan feta.
- o Drizzle with a lemon-oregano vinaigrette.

vi. Mushroom and Spinach Risotto:

- o Sauté mushrooms, spinach, and diced onions in olive oil. Mix with cooked brown rice and vegetable broth.
- o Cook until creamy and top with chopped fresh parsley.

vii. Mediterranean Roasted Vegetable Platter:

- o Roast a variety of colorful vegetables (eggplant, bell peppers, zucchini and cherry tomatoes) with olive oil and herbs.
- o Serve with pita bread, hummus, and a side of quinoa.

viii. Vegan Mediterranean Pizza:

- o Use whole grain pizza crust topped with tomato sauce, artichoke hearts, Kalamata olives, red onion, roasted red peppers, and dairy-free cheese.

ix. Vegan Stuffed Grape Leaves (Dolmas):

- o   Mix cooked quinoa with chopped fresh herbs, diced tomatoes, and minced garlic.
- o   Wrap the mixture in grape leaves, and steam until heated.

x. Chickpea and Spinach Coconut Curry:

- o   Sauté onions, bell peppers, and garlic in coconut oil. Add chickpeas, chopped spinach, and curry spices.
- o   Stir in coconut milk and simmer until flavors meld. Serve over brown rice.

These vibrant and diverse plant-based dishes bring a fusion of Mediterranean ingredients and flavors, catering to a variety of taste preferences and dietary choices.

9.2 Incorporating legumes, tofu, and tempeh into your diet

Legumes, tofu, and tempeh are excellent sources of plant-based protein and can be incorporated into various dishes to create nutritious and flavorful meals. Here are some ideas:

i. Legume Salad:

- o   Make a salad with mixed greens, cooked lentils or chickpeas, diced cucumber, cherry tomatoes, red onion, and a lemon-herb vinaigrette.

o   Top with chopped fresh parsley and crumbled feta or diced avocado.

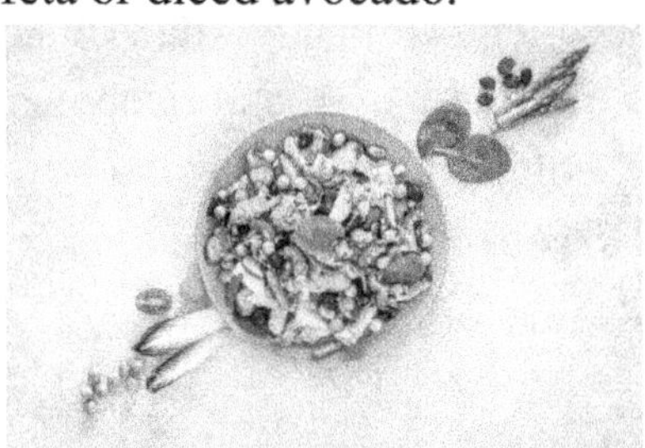

ii. Tofu Stir-Fry:

o   Stir-fry tofu cubes with a mix of colorful vegetables like bell peppers, broccoli, and snap peas.
o   Add a stir-fry sauce made from low-sodium soy sauce, ginger, garlic, and a touch of sesame oil.
o   Serve over brown rice or quinoa.

iii. Chickpea Tacos:

o   Create a taco filling by sautéing cooked chickpeas with taco seasoning, diced tomatoes, and corn.
o   Serve in whole-grain tortillas with shredded lettuce, diced avocado, and a squeeze of lime.

iv. Tempeh Bowl:

- o Marinate sliced tempeh in a mixture of soy sauce, maple syrup, minced garlic, and rice vinegar.
- o Pan-fry until golden and serve over a bowl of mixed greens, cooked quinoa, and roasted vegetables.

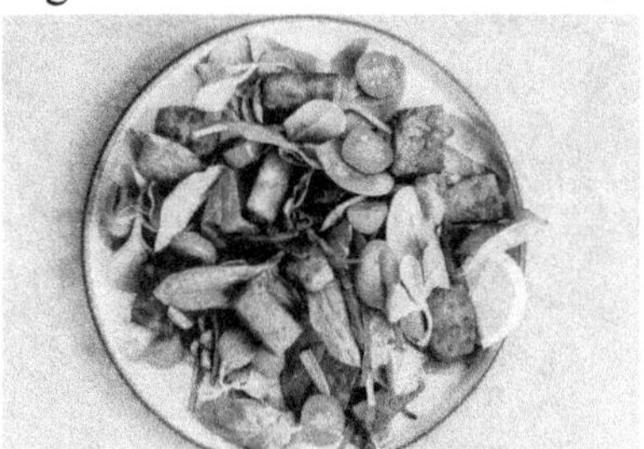

Salad with roasted tempeh, cherry tomato, lettuce, beetroot straws and spinach

v. Lentil Curry:

- o Make a flavorful lentil curry by sautéing onions, bell peppers, and garlic in coconut oil.
- o Add cooked lentils, diced tomatoes, and curry spices. Stir in coconut milk and simmer until well combined.
- o Serve with whole wheat naan or brown rice.

vi. Tofu Scramble:

- o Crumble firm tofu and sauté with diced onions, bell peppers, and spinach.

- o Season with turmeric, nutritional yeast, and a pinch of black salt (for an eggy flavor).
- o Serve with whole-grain toast and avocado slices.

vii. Hummus and Veggie Wrap:

- o Spread hummus on a whole-grain tortilla and fill it with sliced cucumbers, shredded carrots, bell peppers, and mixed greens.
- o Add a sprinkle of toasted sunflower seeds for crunch.

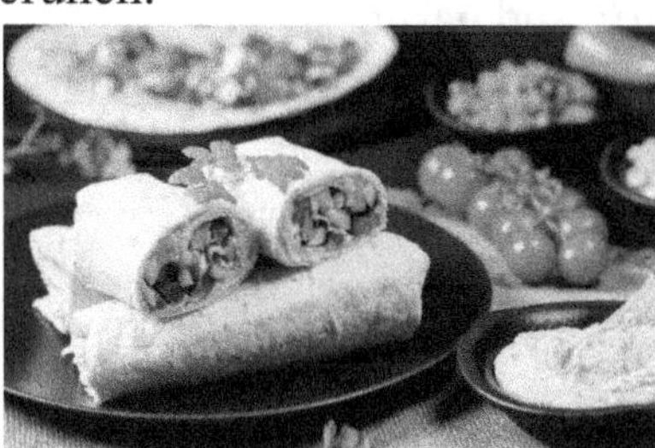

Tortilla with vegetables and hummus with chickpeas

viii. Tempeh Salad Bowl:

- o Combine mixed greens with sliced tempeh, roasted sweet potatoes, quinoa, and a variety of colorful vegetables.
- o Drizzle with a tahini-lemon dressing and top with chopped nuts.

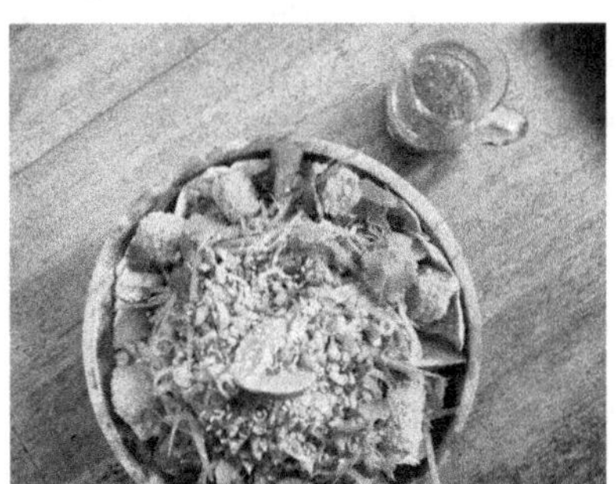

Tempeh noodle salad with peanut dressing

ix. Lentil Soup:

- o Make a hearty lentil soup with sautéed onions, carrots, celery, and garlic.
- o Add cooked lentils, vegetable broth, diced tomatoes, and your favorite herbs and spices.

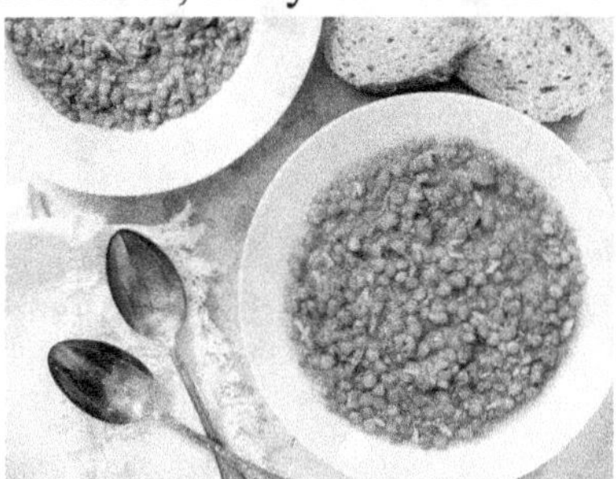

Lentil soup with crusted bread

x. Tofu and Vegetable Skewers:

- o Thread tofu cubes and assorted vegetables onto skewers.

o   Grill or bake until tofu is golden, and vegetables are tender. Serve with a side of whole grain.

These ideas showcase the versatility of legumes, tofu, and tempeh in creating diverse and satisfying plant-based meals that are rich in protein and other essential nutrients.

Chapter 10: Wholesome Whole Grains

Whole grains are a fantastic addition to a balanced and nutritious diet. Here are some wholesome whole-grain options along with ideas on how to incorporate them into your meals:

1. Quinoa:

o   Use quinoa as a base for grain bowls, salads, or stir-fries.

o Make a quinoa and vegetable stuffed bell pepper
or squash.

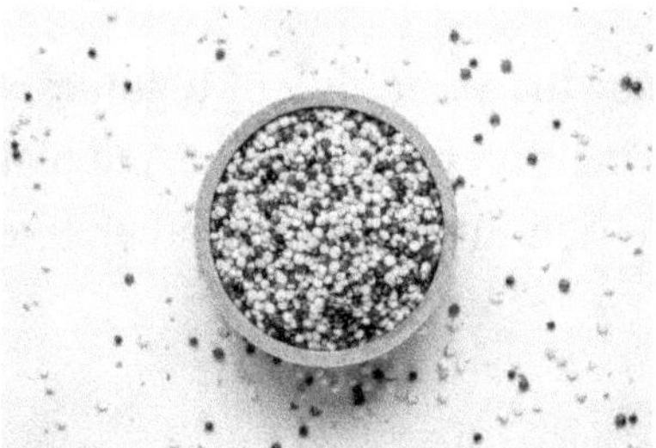

Varieties of uncooked quinoa grains

2. Brown Rice:

o Serve stir-fries or tofu/tempeh bowls over cooked
brown rice.
o Make a vegetable and brown rice casserole.

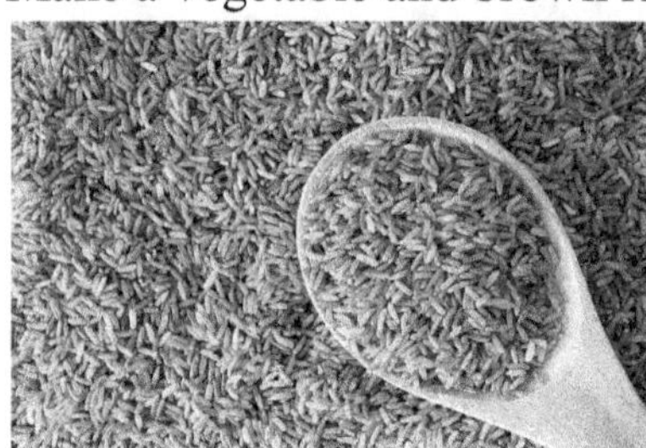

Brown rice grains

3.Whole Wheat Pasta:

o Enjoy pasta dishes with whole wheat pasta and a
variety of vegetables.
o Make a Mediterranean-style pasta salad with
chopped tomatoes, olives, cucumber, and feta.

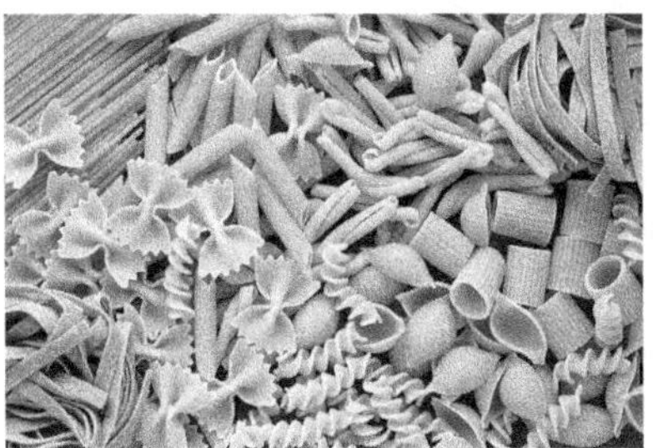

Varieties of whole wheat pasta

4. Farro:

- o Use Farro as a base for warm grain salads with roasted vegetables.
- o Make a farro and vegetable stir-fry.

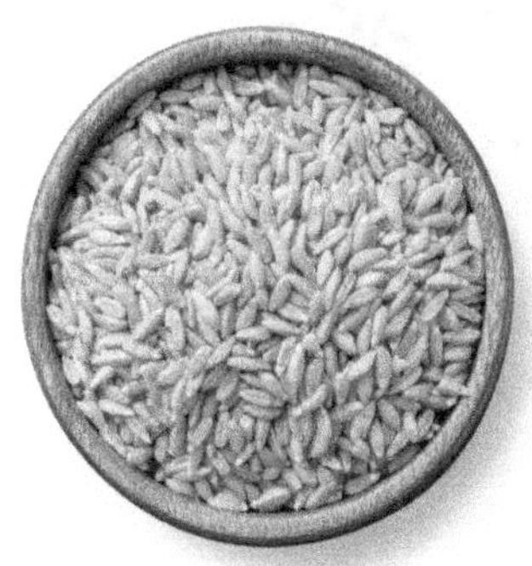

Farro grains

5. Barley:

- o Add cooked barley to soups for extra texture and nutrition.
- o Create a barley and mushroom risotto-style dish.

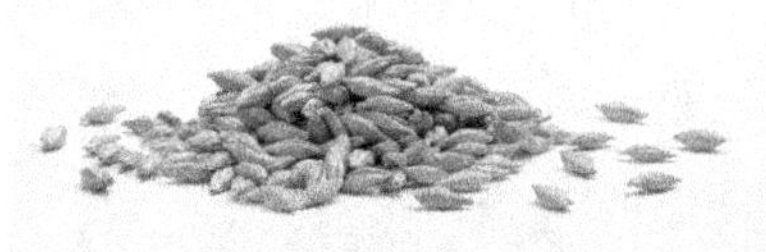

Pile of barley grains

6. Bulgur:

- o Make a hearty tabbouleh salad with chopped vegetables, parsley, lemon juice, and olive oil.
- o Use bulgur in stuffed pepper or stuffed cabbage recipes.

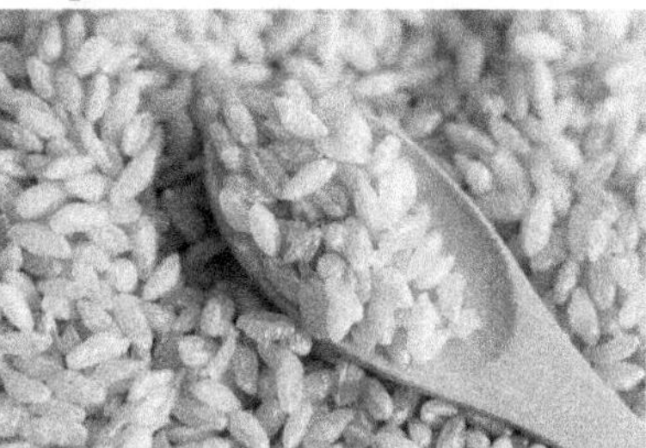

Bulgur, raw wheat grains

7. Millet:

- o Prepare millet porridge for breakfast with your favorite toppings.

o   Use cooked millet as a base for plant-based patties.

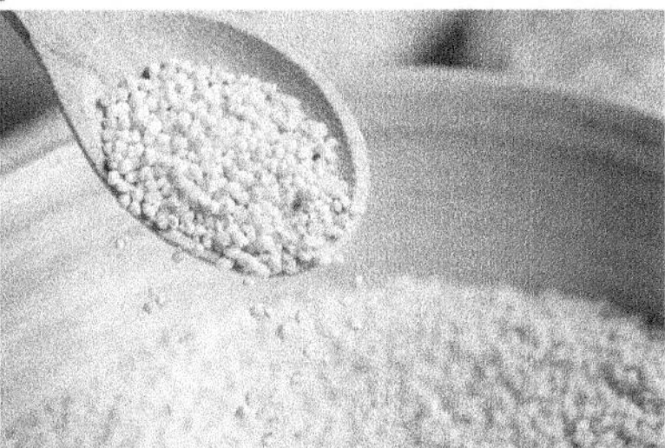

Hulled millet grains

8. Oats:

o   Start your day with a bowl of oatmeal topped with fresh fruit and nuts.
o   Blend oats into smoothies for added fiber and thickness.

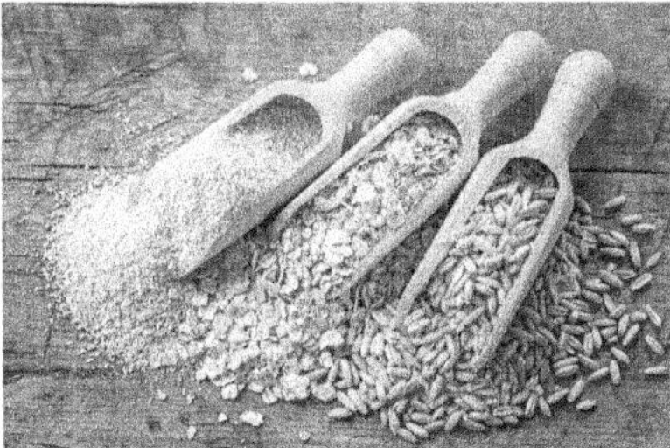

Oat flakes seeds

9. Freekeh:

o   Use freekeh as a base for grain and vegetable bowls.

- o Mix cooked freekeh with chopped herbs, diced vegetables, and a lemon-tahini dressing.

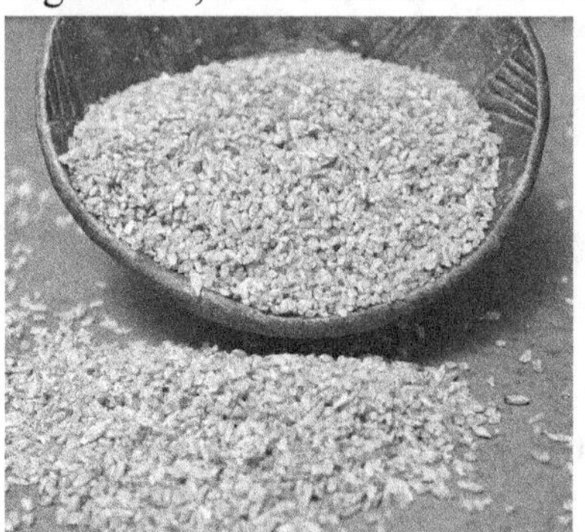

Freekeh grains – an antioxidant

10. Spelt:

- o Cook spelt and use it in grain salads with roasted vegetables and beans.
- o Make a spelt and vegetable stir-fry.

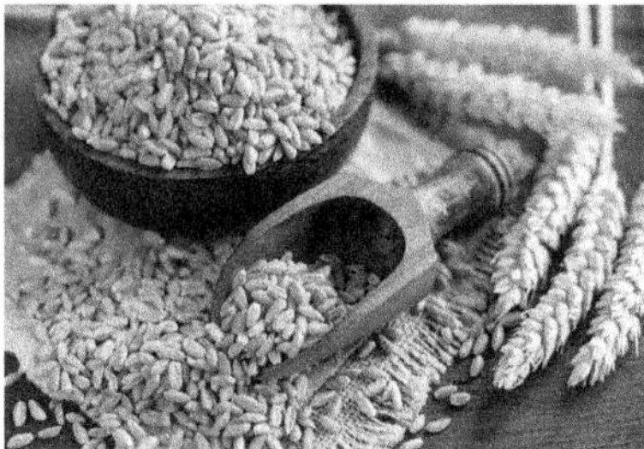

Spelt grains

Remember to pair whole grains with a variety of vegetables, legumes, and plant-based proteins to create well-balanced and nutrient-rich meals that support a healthy diet.

10.1 Discover the wonders of ancient grains and their benefits

Ancient grains are a group of grains that have been cultivated for thousands of years and are regaining popularity due to their nutritional benefits, unique flavors, and versatility. Here are some examples of ancient grains and their benefits:

1. Quinoa:

- Quinoa is a complete protein, containing all essential amino acids.
- It's high in fiber, aiding digestion and promoting a feeling of fullness.
- It is rich in minerals like magnesium, iron, and potassium.

2. Farro:

- Farro is a good source of complex carbohydrates and dietary fiber.
- It contains B vitamins, including niacin and B6, which are important for energy metabolism.

3. Amaranth:

- o Amaranth is high in protein and contains lysine, an amino acid often lacking in other grains.
- o It's gluten-free and a good source of calcium and iron.

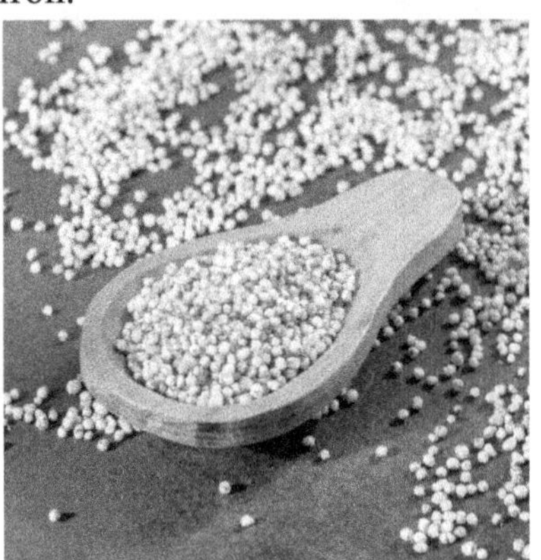

Popped amaranth grains

4. Freekeh:

- o Freekeh is rich in fiber and protein, promoting satiety and digestive health.
- o It contains prebiotics that support gut health.

5. Millet:

- o Millet is gluten-free and easily digestible.
- o It's a good source of magnesium, which supports heart health and relaxation.

6. Spelt:

- o Spelt contains complex carbohydrates and dietary fiber, providing sustained energy.
- o It contains a variety of nutrients including B vitamins, iron, and manganese.

7. Teff:

- o Teff is a great source of iron, which is important for oxygen transport in the body.
- o It is rich in resistant starch, supporting gut health.

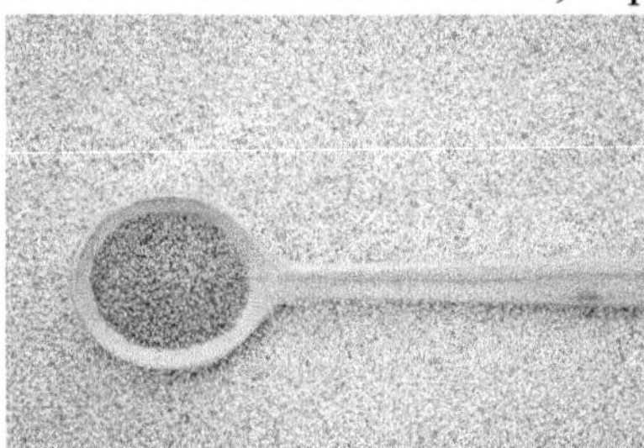

Teff grains

8. Kamut:

- o Kamut has a higher protein content than modern wheat and contains selenium, a powerful antioxidant.
- o It's rich in heart-healthy fats and vitamin E.

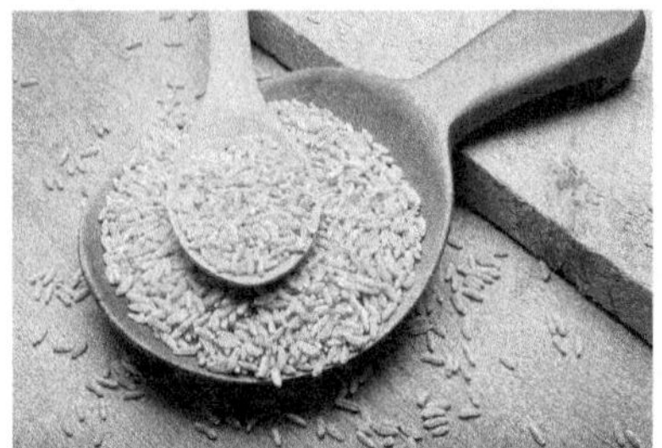

Organic kamut grains

9. Einkorn:

- o Einkorn contains higher levels of protein and essential fatty acids than modern wheat.
- o It's rich in lutein, a carotenoid important for eye health.

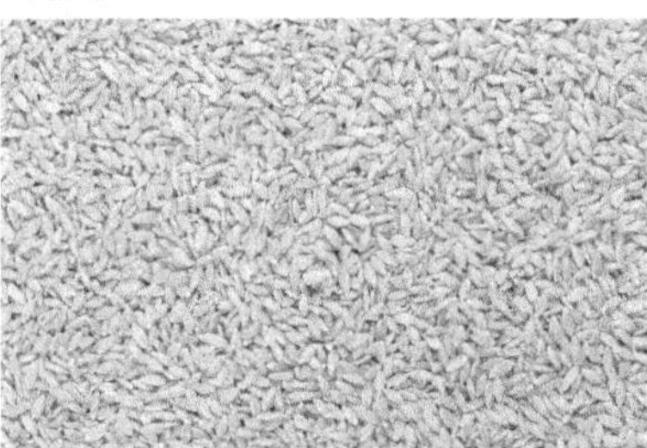

Hulled einkorn wheat grains

10. Sorghum:

- o Sorghum is gluten-free and packed with antioxidants.

o It's rich in magnesium, which supports bone
   health

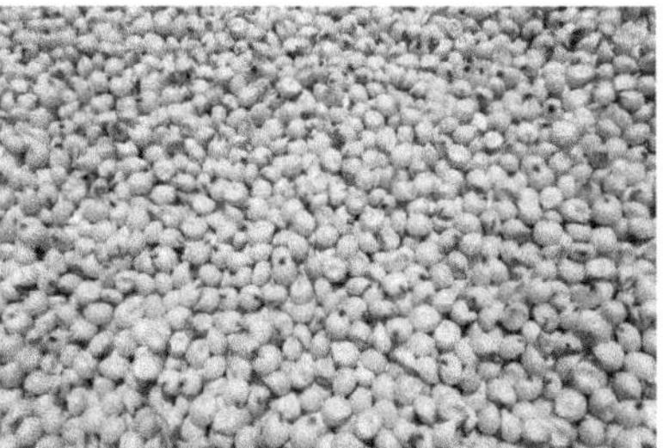

White millet (Sorghum) grains

Ancient grains offer a wide range of nutrients, including
fiber, vitamins, minerals, and antioxidants. They can be
used in a variety of dishes, from salads and grain bowls
to soups and baked goods. Incorporating these grains
into your diet can add diversity, flavor, and a nutrient
boost to your meals.

10.2 Creative Mediterranean grain-based recipes

Here are some creative Mediterranean-inspired grain-
based recipes that highlight the flavors and versatility of
ancient grains:

i. Quinoa Tabbouleh:

o Make a classic tabbouleh salad by combining
   cooked quinoa with chopped fresh parsley, diced
   tomatoes, cucumber, red onion, and fresh mint.

o   Toss with a lemon-olive oil dressing and serve as a refreshing side dish.

ii. Farro Risotto with Roasted Vegetables:

o   Create a creamy farro risotto by sautéing farro with onions and garlic, then gradually adding vegetable broth until cooked.
o   Roast a variety of vegetables (zucchini, bell peppers, cherry tomatoes) and fold them into the risotto along with chopped fresh basil and grated Parmesan.

iii. Amaranth Stuffed Bell Peppers:

o   Cook amaranth and mix with sautéed onions, garlic, spinach, diced tomatoes, and crumbled feta.
o   Stuff the mixture into bell peppers and bake until peppers are tender.

iv. Freekeh Greek Salad:

o   Toss cooked freekeh with diced cucumber, red onion, Kalamata olives, cherry tomatoes, and crumbled vegan feta.

- o Drizzle with a lemon-oregano vinaigrette and sprinkle with chopped fresh dill.

v. Millet and Vegetable Stirry:

- o Stir-fry cooked millet with a mix of colorful vegetables, like broccoli, bell peppers, and snap peas.
- o Add a sauce made from low-sodium soy sauce, ginger, garlic, and sesame oil.

vi. Spelt Mediterranean Bowl:

- o Build a bowl with cooked spelt, roasted chickpeas, grilled eggplant, artichoke hearts, and a variety of fresh vegetables.
- o Drizzle with a tahini-lemon dressing and sprinkle with chopped parsley.

vii. Teff Breakfast Porridge:

- o Cook teff into a creamy porridge with almond milk, cinnamon, and a touch of maple syrup.
- o Top with sliced bananas, chopped nuts, and a drizzle of honey.

viii. Kamut Stuffed Mushrooms:

- o Mix cooked kamut with sautéed mushrooms, garlic, chopped fresh thyme, and vegan cream cheese.

- o   Stuff mushroom caps with the mixture and bake until the mushrooms are tender.

ix. Einkorn Tomato Risotto:

- o   Make a tomato risotto using einkorn by sautéing einkorn with onions and garlic, then adding diced tomatoes and vegetable broth.
- o   Finish with chopped fresh basil and a sprinkle of nutritional yeast.

x. Sorghum Greek Bowl:

- o   Create a grain bowl with cooked sorghum, falafel, diced cucumber, cherry tomatoes, red onions, and a dollop of tzatziki sauce.

These recipes showcase the culinary potential of ancient grains in Mediterranean-inspired dishes, bringing a harmonious blend of flavors, textures, and nutrients to your meals.

Chapter 11: Decadent Desserts (PCOS-Friendly)

Here are some decadent and PCOS-friendly dessert ideas that incorporate wholesome ingredients and mindful choices:

i. Chia Seed Pudding with Berries:

- o Mix chia seeds with almond milk and a touch of vanilla extract.
- o Let it sit in the fridge to thicken overnight. Serve with a medley of fresh berries.

ii, Dark Chocolate-Dipped Strawberries:

- o Dip fresh strawberries in melted dark chocolate (70% cocoa or higher).
- o Let them cool and harden on parchment paper.

iii. Baked Apples with Cinnamon and Nuts:

- o Core apples and stuff them with a mixture of chopped nuts, cinnamon, and a drizzle of honey or maple syrup.
- o Bake until the apples are tender.

iv. Frozen Banana Bites:

- o Slice bananas into bite-sized pieces and dip them in melted dark chocolate.
- o Place them on a parchment-lined tray and freeze until the chocolate is set.

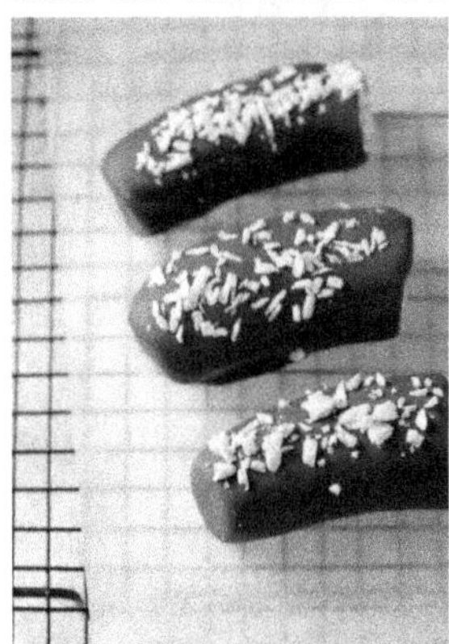

Frozen bananas in dark chocolate with nuts

iv. Greek Yogurt Parfait:

- o Layer plain Greek yogurt with mixed berries, chopped nuts, and a drizzle of honey.

v. Coconut and Almond Energy Balls:

- o Blend dates, almonds, shredded coconut, and a touch of vanilla extract in a food processor.
- o Roll the mixture into small balls and refrigerate until firm.

vi. Berry Sorbet:

- o Blend frozen mixed berries with a splash of almond milk until smooth.
- o Serve immediately as a refreshing sorbet.

vii. Baked Oatmeal Cups:

- o Mix rolled oats, mashed banana, almond milk, chopped nuts, and a sprinkle of cinnamon.
- o Portion the mixture into muffin cups and bake until firm.

viii. Almond Butter and Banana Slices:

- o Spread almond butter on banana slices and sprinkle with chopped nuts or a touch of cinnamon.

ix. Yogurt-Dipped Grapes:

- o Dip red or green grapes in plain Greek yogurt and freeze until the yogurt is firm.

These dessert ideas focus on using natural sweetness from fruits and honey while incorporating nutrient-rich ingredients. Enjoying treats in moderation and choosing whole, unprocessed ingredients can help you create decadent desserts that align with a PCOS-friendly diet.

11.1 Satisfy your sweet tooth with guilt-free treats

Here are some guilt-free sweet treat ideas to satisfy your sweet tooth while keeping things healthy:

a) Fruit Salad with Mint:

- Create a colorful fruit salad with a variety of your favorite fruits.
- Add a touch of chopped fresh mint for extra flavor.

b) Chocolate Avocado Mousse:

- Blend ripe avocado with cocoa powder, a touch of honey or maple syrup, and a splash of almond milk.
- Chill the mixture for a rich and creamy chocolate mousse.

c) Frozen Yogurt Bark:

- Spread plain Greek yogurt on a baking sheet.
- Top with chopped fruits, nuts, and a drizzle of honey. Freeze until firm, then break into pieces.

d) Date and Nut Energy Bites:

- o Blend dates, nuts (like almonds or cashews), a touch of vanilla extract, and a pinch of salt in a food processor.
- o Roll into small balls and refrigerate.

e) Baked Cinnamon Apple Slices:

- o Slice apples and toss them with a sprinkle of cinnamon.
- o Bake until tender and enjoy warm.

f) Chia Seed Pudding Parfait:

- o Mix chia seeds with almond milk and a touch of vanilla. Let it sit to thicken.
- o Layer with mixed berries and chopped nuts for a parfait.

g) Dark Chocolate-Covered Almonds:

- o Dip whole almonds in melted dark chocolate (70% cocoa or higher).
- o Let them cool and harden.

h) Coconut and Berry Popsicles:

- o Blend coconut water with mixed berries and a touch of honey.
- o Pour into popsicle molds and freeze until solid.

i) Baked Banana with Cinnamon and Almonds:

- o Slice a banana lengthwise, sprinkle with cinnamon, and top with chopped almonds.
- o Bake until the banana is soft and toppings are toasted.

j) Rice Cake with Nut Butter and Banana:

- o Spread nut butter on a rice cake and top with banana slices.

These treats offer a balance of natural sweetness, healthy fats, and fiber, making them guilt-free options to satisfy your sweet cravings. Remember, moderation is key, and choosing nutrient-rich ingredients can make your sweet indulgences more enjoyable and beneficial.

11.2 Reduced sugar and healthier dessert options

Here are some reduced sugar and healthier dessert options that still deliver on flavor and satisfaction:

a) Baked Apples with Cinnamon:

- o Core apples and stuff them with a mixture of chopped nuts, raisins, and a sprinkle of cinnamon.

- o Bake until the apples are tender and enjoy warm.

b) Greek Yogurt Parfait with Nuts and Berries:

- o Layer plain Greek yogurt with mixed berries, chopped nuts, and a drizzle of honey or maple syrup.

c) Chocolate-Dipped Banana Bites:

- o Dip banana slices in melted dark chocolate (70% cocoa or higher) and freeze until the chocolate is set.

d) Chia Seed Pudding with Fruit:

- o Mix chia seeds with almond milk and a touch of vanilla extract.
- o Top with sliced fruits like mango, kiwi, or berries.

e) Fruit Sorbet:

- o Blend frozen fruits (such as berries, mango, or pineapple) with a splash of water or almond milk until smooth.
- o Serve immediately for a refreshing sorbet.

f) Coconut Rice Pudding:

- o Make rice pudding using coconut milk, brown rice, and a touch of honey or maple syrup for sweetness.
- o Sprinkle with chopped nuts and a pinch of cinnamon.

g) Oatmeal Banana Cookies:

- o Mash ripe bananas and mix with rolled oats, a pinch of cinnamon, and a handful of dark chocolate chips or dried fruit.
- o Drop spoonfuls onto a baking sheet and bake until golden.

h) Mixed Berry Crumble:

- o Toss mixed berries with a touch of honey or maple syrup and a sprinkle of whole wheat flour.
- o Top with a mixture of oats, chopped nuts, and a touch of coconut oil. Bake until bubbly.

i) Dark Chocolate-Dipped Strawberries:

- o Dip fresh strawberries in melted dark chocolate (70% cocoa or higher).
- o Allow them to cool and harden on parchment paper.

j) Fruit Salad with Honey-Lime Dressing:

- o Toss together a variety of fresh fruits and drizzle with a dressing made from honey and lime juice.

These dessert options prioritize whole ingredients and natural sweetness, offering you healthier choices while still enjoying delicious treats.

Chapter 12: Hydration and Refreshments

Staying hydrated is important for overall well-being. Here are some refreshing hydration options:

i. Infused Water:

- o Create your own flavored water by infusing it with slices of citrus fruits, cucumber, mint, or berries.

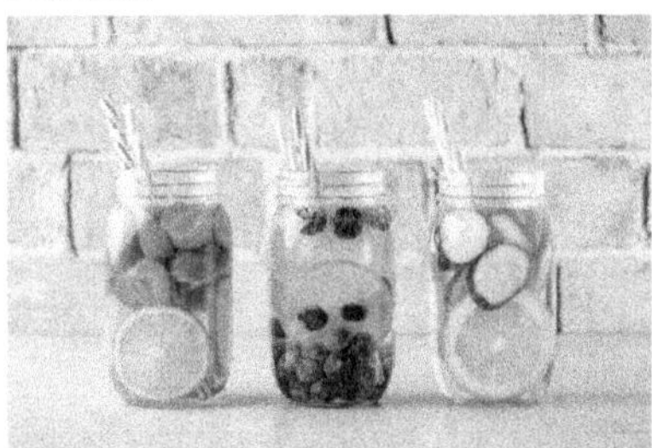

Healthy detox infused water

ii. Herbal Iced Tea:

- o Brew herbal teas like chamomile, peppermint, or hibiscus and chill them for a refreshing beverage.

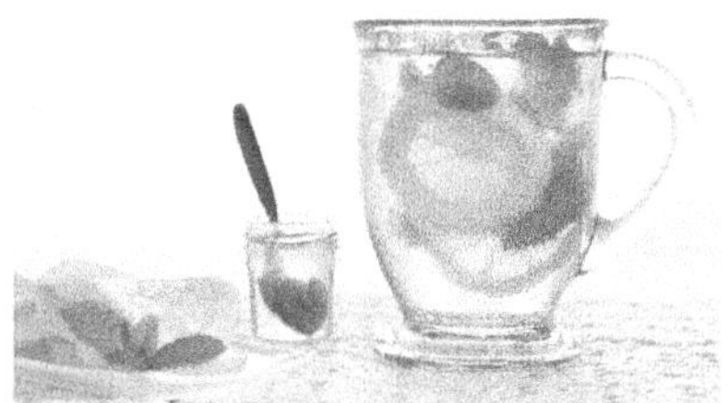

Ice tea with lemonade

iii. Coconut Water:

- o Enjoy the natural electrolytes in coconut water for a hydrating boost.

iv. Cucumber-Mint Cooler:

- o Blend cucumber, mint leaves, and a splash of lime juice with water or coconut water for a cooling drink.

v. Sparkling Water with Citrus:

- o Mix sparkling water with a squeeze of lemon, lime, or orange for a fizzy, refreshing option.

vi. Homemade Lemonade:

o   Make your own lemonade using freshly squeezed
lemon juice, water, and a touch of honey or a
natural sweetener.

vii. Watermelon Slushie:

o   Blend watermelon chunks with ice for a
hydrating and naturally sweet slushie.

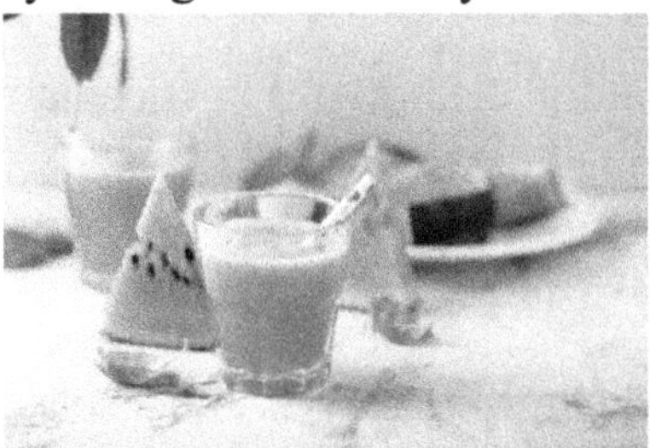

Watermelon drink

viii. Iced Green Tea:

o   Brew green tea, let it cool, and serve over ice
with a hint of lemon or honey.

ix. Berry Smoothie:

o   Blend mixed berries with water, a splash of
almond milk, or coconut water for a hydrating
and antioxidant-rich drink.

x. Homemade Electrolyte Drink:

- o Mix water, a pinch of sea salt, a touch of honey, and a squeeze of lemon for a DIY electrolyte drink.

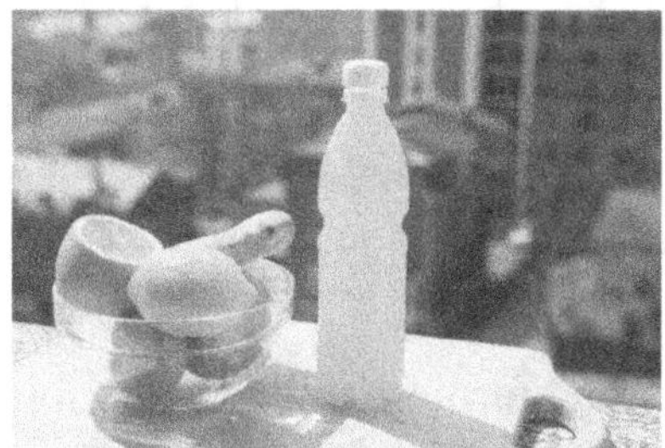

Homemade isotonic drink

Remember to listen to your body's thirst cues and aim to consume a variety of hydrating beverages throughout the day to maintain proper hydration levels.

12.1 Nourishing beverages inspired by the Mediterranean region

The Mediterranean region is known for its refreshing and nourishing beverages. Here are some beverages inspired by the Mediterranean that you might enjoy:

i. Mint Lemonade:

- o Make a classic lemonade with freshly squeezed lemon juice and water.

o   Add a handful of fresh mint leaves and a touch of honey for sweetness.

ii. Iced Herbal Tea with Citrus:

o   Brew herbal teas like chamomile, rosemary, or thyme, and let them cool.
o   Serve over ice with a slice of orange or lemon.

iii. Turmeric Golden Milk:

o   Make a warming turmeric milk by mixing almond milk with turmeric, cinnamon, and a touch of honey.
o   Heat it gently or serve it chilled.

iv. Greek Frappé Coffee:

o   Mix instant coffee with water and sugar, if desired.
o   Shake or blend until frothy and serve over ice.

v. Tamarind Juice:

o   Create tamarind juice by dissolving tamarind paste in water and adding a touch of honey or agave for sweetness.
o   Serve chilled.

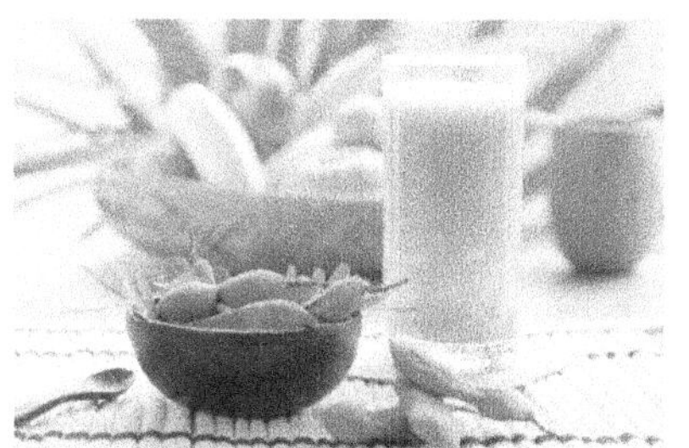

Tamarind composition

vi. Hibiscus Iced Tea:

- o Brew hibiscus tea and let it cool. Add a touch of honey or maple syrup for sweetness.
- o Serve over ice with a slice of lemon.

vii. Cucumber-Lemon Water:

- o Infuse water with slices of cucumber and lemon for a refreshing and hydrating drink

viii. Pomegranate Sparkler:

- o Mix pomegranate juice with sparkling water and add a squeeze of lime juice.
- o Serve over ice with a sprig of mint.

ix. Orange Blossom Water Spritzer:

- o Mix a few drops of orange blossom water with still or sparkling water.
- o Add a twist of orange peel for extra flavor.

x. Rosemary Citrus Cooler:

- o Muddle fresh rosemary with lemon and orange slices.
- o Mix with water and a touch of honey, and serve over ice.

These Mediterranean-inspired beverages offer a blend of flavors and ingredients that are not only refreshing but also carry some of the distinctive tastes of the region.

12.2 Infused waters, herbal teas, and mocktails

Here's a collection of infused waters, herbal teas, and mocktails to help you stay refreshed and hydrated:

1. Infused Waters:

a) Citrus Mint Infused Water:

- o Combine slices of lemon, lime, and fresh mint leaves in a pitcher of water. Let it infuse in the fridge.

b) Cucumber and Basil Infused Water:

- o Add cucumber slices and a few basil leaves to the water for a cooling and aromatic drink.

c) Berry Blast Infused Water:

- o Drop a handful of mixed berries (strawberries, blueberries, raspberries) into the water for a burst of fruity flavor.

d) Ginger and Lemon Infused Water:

- o Add thin slices of fresh ginger and lemon to water for a zesty and invigorating infusion.

2. Herbal Teas:

a) Chamomile Lavender Tea:

- o Brew chamomile tea and add a sprinkle of dried lavender flowers for a soothing and calming blend.

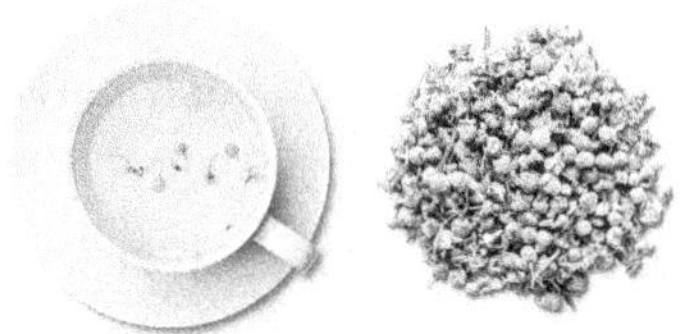

A cup of chamomile and lavender tea

b) Mint Verbena Tea:

- o Combine mint leaves and lemon verbena leaves for a refreshing herbal tea.

c) Rosehip Hibiscus Tea:

    o   Brew rosehip and hibiscus tea for a tart and vibrant infusion packed with vitamin C.

d) Lemon-Ginger Herbal Tea:

    o   Make tea with fresh ginger slices and a squeeze of lemon. Add honey for sweetness.

3. Mocktails:

a) Virgin Mojito:

    o   Muddle fresh mint leaves and lime wedges with a touch of sugar or honey.
    o   Top with soda water and crushed ice.

b) Sparkling Basil Lemonade:

    o   Mix fresh lemon juice, a few basil leaves, and a touch of agave or honey.
    o   Add sparkling water and serve over ice.

c) Cranberry Ginger Fizz:

    o   Mix cranberry juice, a splash of ginger syrup, and soda water.
    o   Garnish with a twist of lime.

d) Pineapple Mint Mocktail:

- o   Blend fresh pineapple chunks with mint leaves and a bit of coconut water.
- o   Strain and serve the refreshing mixture over ice.

These infused waters, herbal teas, and mocktails offer a variety of flavors and options to keep you hydrated and satisfied, whether you're looking for something subtle, soothing, or delightfully zesty.

Chapter 13: Weekly Meal Plans And Shopping Lists

Here's a sample Mediterranean-inspired weekly meal plan along with a corresponding shopping list to get you started:

1. Weekly Meal Plan:

- **Day 1**:

- **Breakfast**: Greek yogurt with mixed berries and chopped nuts.

- **Lunch**: Quinoa salad with cucumbers, tomatoes, red onion, Kalamata olives, feta, and lemon-herb vinaigrette.

- **Dinner**: Grilled chicken or tofu with roasted vegetables and a side of whole wheat pita.

- **Day 2**:

- **Breakfast**: Whole grain toast with smashed avocado and a sprinkle of feta.

- **Lunch**: Chickpea salad with diced bell peppers, red onion, parsley, lemon juice, and olive oil.

- **Dinner**: Baked salmon with quinoa and steamed broccoli.

- **Day 3**:

- **Breakfast**: Smoothie with spinach, banana, mixed berries, almond milk, and a scoop of protein powder.

- **Lunch**: Greek salad with romaine lettuce, tomatoes, cucumber, red onion, olives, and feta.

- **Dinner**: Lentil soup with a side of whole grain bread.

- **Day 4**:

- **Breakkfast**: Oatmeal with sliced banana, chopped nuts, and a drizzle of honey.

- **Lunch**: Whole grain wrap with hummus, roasted vegetables, and a sprinkle of feta.

- **Dinner**: Stuffed bell peppers with brown rice, black beans, corn, tomatoes, and spices.

- **Day 5**:

- **Breakfast**: Scrambled eggs or tofu with sautéed spinach and cherry tomatoes.

- **Lunch**: Farro salad with diced cucumber, mint, parsley, red onion, and lemon-tahini dressing.

- **Dinner**: Whole wheat pasta with marinara sauce, grilled eggplant, and a side salad.

- **Day 6**:

- **Breakfast**: Greek yogurt parfait with granola and mixed berries.

- **Lunch**: Quinoa and black bean bowl with avocado, salsa, and a dollop of Greek yogurt.

- **Dinner**: Grilled vegetable kebabs with herbed couscous.

- **Day 7**:

- **Breakfast**: Smoothie with mixed berries, banana, almond milk, spinach, and a spoonful of almond butter.

- **Lunch**: Mediterranean-style sandwich with whole grain bread, hummus, roasted red peppers, spinach, and olives.

- **Dinner**: Baked falafel with tabbouleh and a side of pita bread.

2. Shopping List:

- Greek yogurt
- Mixed berries (fresh or frozen)

- Mixed vegetables for salads and cooking (tomatoes, cucumbers, bell peppers, red onion, spinach, etc.)
- Whole grains (quinoa, brown rice, whole wheat pasta, farro)
- Protein sources (chicken, tofu, salmon, eggs, lentils, black beans, chickpeas)
- Nuts and seeds (chopped nuts, almond butter)
- Feta cheese
- Hummus
- Olives (Kalamata or green)
- Olive oil
- Lemon
- Fresh herbs (mint, parsley, basil)
- Whole grain bread and pita
- Whole grain wraps
- Avocado
- Spices (cumin, paprika, oregano, etc.)
- Almond milk
- Smoothie ingredients (banana, spinach, mixed berries)
- Nutritional staples (honey, tahini)
- Vegetables for roasting and grilling (zucchini, eggplant, broccoli, etc.)

Feel free to adjust portion sizes and ingredients based on your preferences and dietary needs. This meal plan and shopping list can serve as a starting point for your Mediterranean-inspired week of meals!

13.1 Convenient meal plans tailored for PCOS support

Here's a sample convenient meal plan tailored for PCOS support. This plan focuses on balanced meals with PCOS-friendly ingredients:

- **Day 1:**

- **Breakfast**: Greek yogurt with mixed berries and a sprinkle of chopped almonds.

- **Lunch**: Spinach salad with grilled chicken, cherry tomatoes, cucumbers, and a light balsamic vinaigrette.

- **Snack**: Carrot sticks with hummus.

- **Dinner**: Baked salmon with quinoa and roasted broccoli.

- **Day 2:**

- **Breakfast**: Oatmeal topped with sliced banana, chia seeds, and a drizzle of honey.

- **Lunch**: Chickpea and vegetable stir-fry with brown rice.

- **Snack**: Apple slices with almond butter.

- **Dinner**: Lentil soup with a side of whole grain bread and a mixed green salad.

- **Day 3:**

- **Breakfast**: Smoothie with spinach, mixed berries, almond milk, and a scoop of protein powder.

- **Lunch**: Mediterranean-style wrap with hummus, grilled vegetables, and feta in a whole grain tortilla.

- **Snack**: Handful of mixed nuts.

- **Dinner**: Grilled turkey burger with a side salad and quinoa.

- **Day 4:**

- **Breakfast**: Scrambled eggs with sautéed spinach and tomatoes.

- **Lunch**: Quinoa salad with black beans, corn, red onion, and a lemon-tahini dressing.

- **Snack**: Greek yogurt with a drizzle of honey.

- **Dinner**: Stir-fried tofu with broccoli and brown rice.

- **Day 5:**

- **Breakfast**: Whole grain toast with avocado and a sprinkle of red pepper flakes.

- **Lunch**: Greek salad with mixed greens, olives, cucumber, red onion, and grilled chicken.

- **Snack**: Celery sticks with almond butter.

- **Dinner**: Baked fish with roasted Brussels sprouts and a side of sweet potato.

- **Day 6:**

- **Breakfast**: Chia seed pudding made with almond milk, topped with fresh berries.

- **Lunch**: Turkey and vegetable wrap in a whole grain tortilla, with a side of carrot sticks.

- **Snack**: Cottage cheese with sliced peaches.

- **Dinner**: Lentil and vegetable curry served over brown rice.

- **Day 7:**

- **Breakfast**: Smoothie with kale, pineapple, almond milk, and a scoop of protein powder.

- **Lunch**: Quinoa and roasted vegetable bowl with a tahini dressing.

- **Snack**: Edamame beans.

- **Dinner**: Grilled chicken breast with steamed broccoli and quinoa.

Remember to adjust portion sizes and ingredients according to your individual needs. This meal plan provides a variety of nutrients and includes PCOS-friendly foods to support your health and well-being.

13.2 Comprehensive shopping lists for each plan

Here are comprehensive shopping lists corresponding to the two meal plans mentioned earlier:

1. Shopping List For a Mediterranean-Inspired Weekly Meal Plan:

i. Proteins:

- Chicken (breast or thighs)
- Salmon
- Eggs
- Tofu

- Falafel (ready-made or ingredients to make your own)
- Ground turkey

ii. Grains:

- Quinoa
- Whole wheat pasta
- Whole grain bread
- Whole wheat wraps or tortillas
- Brown rice
- Whole wheat pita

iii. Fruits and Vegetables:

- Mixed berries (fresh or frozen)
- Lemons
- Limes
- Avocado
- Cherry tomatoes
- Cucumbers
- Red onion
- Bell peppers
- Spinach
- Romaine lettuce
- Zucchini
- Eggplant
- Broccoli
- Fresh herbs (mint, parsley and basil)

- Mixed greens for salads
- Apples
- Bananas

iv. Dairy and Dairy Alternatives:

- Greek yogurt
- Almond milk

v. Pantry Staples:

- Olive oil
- Balsamic vinegar
- Hummus
- Mixed nuts (almonds, cashews, etc.)
- Chopped nuts (almonds, walnuts)
- Honey
- Tahini
- Cumin
- Paprika
- Oregano
- Whole grain flour (for baking)

2. Shopping List for a Convenient PCOS Support Meal Plan:

i. Proteins:

- Chicken (breast or thighs)
- Salmon
- Turkey
- Tofu
- Eggs

ii. Grains:

- Quinoa
- Oats
- Whole- grain bread
- Brown rice

iii. Fruits and Vegetables:

- Mixed berries (fresh or frozen)
- Bananas
- Spinach
- Tomatoes
- Broccoli
- Sweet potatoes
- Carrots
- Celery
- Peaches
- Kale
- Pineapple

iv. Dairy and Dairy Alternatives:

- Greek yogurt

- Almond milk
- Cottage cheese

v. Pantry Staples:

- Chia seeds
- Almond butter
- Mixed nuts (almonds, cashews, etc.)
- Honey
- Lemon-tahini dressing
- Olive oil
- Red pepper flakes
- Whole grain flour (for baking)
- Protein powder

Please adjust the quantities based on your personal needs and preferences. These shopping lists cover a range of foods to help you prepare the meals outlined in the meal plans.

Chapter 14: Lifestyle Tips For PCOS Management

Managing PCOS involves a holistic approach that combines dietary choices, physical activity, stress management, and self-care. Here are some lifestyle tips to support PCOS management:

1. Balanced Diet:

- Focus on a balanced diet rich in whole foods, lean proteins, healthy fats, and complex carbohydrates.
- Choose high-fiber foods like vegetables, fruits, whole grains, and legumes to help stabilize blood sugar levels.

2. Regular Meals:

- Aim for regular meals and snacks to prevent blood sugar spikes and crashes.
- Avoid skipping meals, as this can lead to overeating later.

3. Low -Glycemic -Index Foods:

- Choose foods with a low- glycemic -index (GI) to help regulate blood sugar levels. These include whole grains, legumes, and non-starchy vegetables.

4. Hydration:

- Drink plenty of water throughout the day to stay hydrated and support metabolism.

5. Physical Activity:

- Engage in regular physical activity to improve insulin sensitivity and overall health.
- Aim for a mix of cardiovascular exercise, strength training, and flexibility exercises.

6. Stress Management:

- Practice stress-reduction techniques such as deep breathing, meditation, yoga, or mindfulness.

- Chronic stress can worsen PCOS symptoms, so finding effective stress management strategies is important.

7. Sleep Quality:

- Prioritize good sleep hygiene by aiming for 7-9 hours of quality sleep each night.
- Adequate sleep can positively impact hormonal balance and overall well-being.

8. Weight Management:

- Maintain a healthy weight, as excess weight can exacerbate PCOS symptoms.
- Focus on sustainable changes rather than extreme diets.

9. Mindful Eating:

- Practice mindful eating by paying attention to hunger and fullness cues.
- This can help prevent overeating and promote a healthy relationship with food.

10. Limit Processed Foods:

- Minimize consumption of processed foods high in added sugars, trans fats, and refined carbohydrates.

11. Omega-3 Fatty Acids:

- Include sources of omega-3 fatty acids such as fatty fish (salmon, mackerel) or flaxseeds to support inflammation and hormone balance.

12. Herbal Teas:

- Herbal teas like spearmint tea may help reduce androgen levels in women with PCOS.

13. Regular Check-Ups:

- Schedule regular check-ups with your healthcare provider to monitor your health and PCOS management.

14. Support Network:

- Connect with friends, family, or support groups to share experiences and seek advice.

Remember that everyone's body is unique, so it's important to work with a healthcare provider or registered dietitian who specializes in PCOS management to tailor your lifestyle changes to your specific needs and goals.

14.1 Exercise and stress-reduction techniques

Both exercise and stress-reduction techniques play important roles in managing PCOS. Here's a breakdown of how to incorporate these into your routine:

1. Exercise:

Regular physical activity can help improve insulin sensitivity, manage weight, and boost overall well-being for individuals with PCOS. Aim for a mix of cardiovascular exercise, strength training, and flexibility exercises:

i. Cardiovascular Exercise:

- ✓ Engage in activities like brisk walking, jogging, cycling, swimming, or dancing.
- ✓ Aim for at least 150 minutes of moderate-intensity aerobic exercise per week.

ii. Strength Training:

- ✓ Incorporate strength training exercises using body weight, resistance bands, or weights.

✓ Focus on major muscle groups with exercises like squats, lunges, push-ups, and rows.

iii. Flexibility Exercises:

✓ Include stretching or yoga to improve flexibility and reduce muscle tension.
✓ These exercises can also help with stress reduction.

2. Stress-Reduction Techniques:

Managing stress is crucial for PCOS management, as stress can exacerbate symptoms. Try these stress-reduction techniques:

i. Deep Breathing: Practice deep breathing exercises to trigger the relaxation response. Inhale deeply through your nose, hold for a few seconds, and exhale slowly through your mouth.

ii. Meditation: Set aside time for meditation to clear your mind and reduce stress. Focus on your breath or use guided meditation apps.

iii. Yoga: Engage in yoga sessions that combine gentle movement, stretching, and deep breathing. Yoga can help alleviate stress and promote relaxation.

iv. Mindfulness: Practice mindfulness by being fully present in the moment. This can be done during daily activities like eating, walking, or even washing dishes.

v. Progressive Muscle Relaxation: Tense and relax different muscle groups to release physical tension and promote relaxation.

vi. Journaling: Write in a journal to express your thoughts and emotions. This can help you process feelings and reduce stress.

vii. Social Support: Connect with friends, family, or support groups. Sharing experiences and talking about your feelings can be therapeutic.

viii. Time Management: Plan and prioritize your tasks to reduce feelings of being overwhelmed. Break tasks into smaller steps.

ix. Hobbies: Engage in activities you enjoy, whether it's painting, playing a musical instrument, gardening, or cooking.

x. Professional Help: Consider seeing a mental health professional for techniques tailored to your needs.

Remember, it's important to find what works best for you. Combining regular exercise with stress-reduction techniques can create a comprehensive approach to managing PCOS and promoting overall well-being.

14.2 Practical lifestyle changes to complement the diet

Practical lifestyle changes can greatly complement your PCOS-friendly diet and contribute to better overall health. Here are some practical suggestions to consider:

1. Portion Control: Pay attention to portion sizes to avoid overeating. Use smaller plates and bowls to help control portions.

2. Regular Meals: Aim for regular meal times to maintain stable blood sugar levels. Avoid skipping meals or going long periods without eating.

3. Meal Planning: Plan your meals and snacks ahead of time to avoid making impulsive food choices. This can help you stick to your PCOS-friendly diet.

4. Balanced Snacks: Keep healthy snacks on hand, such as nuts, seeds, Greek yogurt, and cut-up vegetables, to prevent reaching for less nutritious options.

5. Mindful Eating: Practice mindful eating by eating slowly, savoring each bite, and paying attention to hunger and fullness cues.

6. Cooking at Home: Prepare meals at home whenever possible. This allows you to control ingredients and cooking methods.

7. Limit Processed Foods: Minimize consumption of processed foods, sugary snacks, and sugary beverages.

8. Hydration: Drink plenty of water throughout the day. Herbal teas, infused water, and water-rich foods like fruits and vegetables are great options.

9. Sleep Routine: Prioritize sleep by establishing a regular sleep routine. Aim for 7-9 hours of quality sleep each night.

10. Regular Physical Activity: Incorporate exercise into your routine. Choose activities you enjoy to make them sustainable and engaging.

11. Stress Management: Find stress-relief techniques that work for you, such as deep breathing, meditation, yoga, or spending time in nature.

12. Social Support: Connect with friends, family, or support groups. Sharing experiences and challenges can provide emotional support.

13. Hobbies: Engage in hobbies or activities you love to help reduce stress and promote a sense of well-being.

14. Time Management: Organize your schedule to reduce stress and create time for self-care activities.

15. Positive Self-Talk: Cultivate positive self-talk and self-compassion. Be kind to yourself and focus on your progress.

16. Tracking Progress: Keep a journal to track your diet, exercise, mood, and any symptoms. This can help you identify patterns and improvements.

17. Seeking Professional Guidance: Consider working with a registered dietitian or healthcare professional experienced in PCOS management. They can provide personalized guidance and support.

Remember that making gradual changes and finding what works best for you is key. Small lifestyle adjustments can lead to significant improvements in your overall health and well-being when combined with a PCOS-friendly diet.

Appendix: PCOS-Friendly Food Swaps

 Here's an appendix of PCOS-friendly food swaps that you can use to make healthier choices in your diet:

1. Carbohydrates:

- Swap refined grains (white bread and white rice) for whole grains (whole wheat bread, brown rice and quinoa).
- Choose complex carbohydrates with a lower glycemic index to help stabilize blood sugar levels.

2. Fats:

- Opt for healthy fats like avocados, nuts, seeds, and olive oil instead of saturated and trans fats.
- Use olive oil or avocado oil for cooking and as salad dressings.

3. Protein:

- Choose lean sources of protein such as skinless poultry, fish, tofu, legumes, and beans.
- Limit the consumption of red and processed meats.

4. Dairy:

- Consider alternatives like almond milk, coconut milk, or lactose-free dairy if you're sensitive to regular cow's milk.
- Choose plain Greek yogurt over sugary- flavored yogurts.

5. Sweeteners:

- Use natural sweeteners like honey or maple syrup
  in moderation instead of refined sugars.
- Experiment with stevia, a natural sweetener with
  a lower impact on blood sugar.

6. Snacks:

- Opt for whole fruits, vegetables with hummus, or
  a small handful of nuts as snacks instead of
  processed snacks.
- Choose air-popped popcorn or whole-grain
  crackers for a crunchy option.

7. Beverages:

- Drink water, herbal teas, or infused water instead
  of sugary beverages.
- If you drink coffee, do so in moderation and
  without excessive added sugars.

8. Cooking Methods:

- Choose baking, grilling, steaming, or sautéing
  over deep frying.
- Use herbs, spices, and citrus for flavoring instead
  of heavy sauces.

9. Processed Foods:

- Minimize or avoid heavily processed foods like
  sugary cereals, packaged snacks, and fast food.

- Opt for whole, minimally processed foods as much as possible.

10. Sodium:

- Reduce salt intake by using herbs, spices, and lemon juice for seasoning.
- Be mindful of hidden sources of sodium in processed foods.

11. Fiber:

- Increase fiber intake with whole fruits, vegetables, whole grains, and legumes.
- Fiber helps regulate blood sugar and supports digestive health.

Remember, small changes over time can lead to significant improvements in your diet and overall health. Focus on making sustainable swaps that align with your personal preferences and needs.

A handy reference for replacing ingredients in other recipes

Here's a handy reference guide for replacing ingredients in recipes to make them more PCOS-friendly:

1. Flour:

- Replace white flour with whole wheat flour, almond flour, or oat flour for added fiber and nutrients.

2. Sugar:

- Use natural sweeteners like honey, maple syrup, or stevia instead of refined sugars.
- Reduce the amount of sugar called for in recipes or use fruit purees as a sweetener.

3. Cooking Oils:

- Replace unhealthy oils with olive oil, avocado oil, or coconut oil for cooking and baking.

4. Dairy:

- Substitute dairy milk with almond milk, coconut milk, or lactose-free dairy if needed.
- Use plain Greek yogurt instead of sour cream or heavy cream in recipes.

5. Eggs:

- Use flaxseed or chia seeds mixed with water as an egg substitute in baking (1 tbsp ground seeds + 3 tbsp water per egg).
- Try silken tofu as an egg alternative in creamy dishes.

6. Meats:

- Choose lean proteins like skinless poultry, fish, tofu, or legumes instead of red or processed meats.

7. Pasta and Grains:

- Opt for whole-grain pasta and brown rice instead of refined pasta and white rice.

8. Condiments and Sauces:

- Make homemade dressings with olive oil, vinegar, and herbs instead of store-bought dressings high in sugar and unhealthy fats.
- Replace sugary sauces with homemade tomato-based sauces flavored with herbs and spices.

9. Snacks and Sides:

- Swap chips and processed snacks with fresh fruit, vegetables with hummus, or a handful of nuts.
- Choose air-popped popcorn or whole-grain crackers as a crunchy snack.

10. Baking:

- Experiment with applesauce or mashed bananas as a fat substitute in baked goods.

- Incorporate nuts, seeds, or dried fruits for added texture and flavor.

11. Beverages:

- Drink water, herbal teas, or infused water instead of sugary sodas and juices.

12. Flavoring:

- Use herbs, spices, and citrus for flavoring instead of heavy sauces and excessive salt.
- Try fresh herbs like basil, mint, and cilantro to enhance dishes.

13. Sodium:

- Reduce salt intake by using herbs, spices, and lemon juice for seasoning.
- Be mindful of hidden sources of sodium in processed foods.

Remember, you can get creative with ingredient substitutions to make recipes more PCOS-friendly. Experiment with different options to find what works best for your taste and dietary preferences.

Making any dish PCOS-friendly with simple swaps

Here's a guide on how to make any dish PCOS-friendly with simple ingredient swaps:

1. Carbohydrates:

- Swap white rice, pasta, or bread for whole-grain alternatives like brown rice, whole wheat pasta, or whole-grain bread.

2. Fats:

- Replace butter with olive oil or avocado oil for cooking and baking.

3. Proteins:

- Opt for lean protein sources like skinless chicken, turkey, fish, tofu, or legumes.

4. Dairy:

- Choose lactose-free dairy or dairy alternatives like almond milk, coconut milk, or plain Greek yogurt.

5. Sweeteners:

- Use natural sweeteners like honey, maple syrup, or stevia instead of refined sugars.

6. Snacks:

- Swap processed snacks with whole food options like fruits, vegetables with hummus, or a handful of nuts.

7. Sauces and Dressings:

- Make your own sauces and dressings using olive oil, vinegar, herbs, and spices instead of store-bought versions with added sugars and unhealthy fats.

8. Fried Foods:

- Opt for baked, grilled, or sautéed options instead of fried foods.

9. Baking:

- Experiment with using almond flour, coconut flour, or oats in place of regular flour in baking recipes.

10. Salt:

- Use herbs, spices, and citrus to season dishes
  instead of excessive salt.

11. Fiber:

- Add extra fiber by including vegetables, fruits,
  whole grains, and legumes in your dishes.

12. Portion Control:

- Be mindful of portion sizes to avoid overeating.

13. Processed Foods:

- Minimize or avoid heavily processed foods high
  in sugar, unhealthy fats, and additives.

14. Hydration:

- Drink plenty of water throughout the day and opt
  for water or herbal teas instead of sugary
  beverages.

15. Balanced Meals:

- Aim for balanced meals that include a mix of
  protein, healthy fats, and fiber-rich
  carbohydrates.

Remember, the key is to focus on whole, nutrient-dense
foods and make simple swaps that align with your
PCOS-friendly dietary goals. These swaps can help you

enjoy a wide variety of dishes while supporting your
health and well-being.